EDUCATION IN A COMPETITIVE AND GLOBALIZING WORLD

TIME OUT: EXAMINING SECLUSION AND RESTRAINT IN SCHOOLS

LAURA E. KENTLEY
EDITOR

Nova Science Publishers, Inc.
New York

For permission to use material from this book please contact us:
Telephone 631-231-7269; Fax 631-231-8175
Web Site: http://www.novapublishers.com

LIBRARY OF CONGRESS CATALOGING-IN-PUBLICATION DATA

Time out : examining seclusion and restraint in schools / editor, Laura E. Kentley.
p. cm.
Includes index.
ISBN 978-1-60876-932-2 (hardcover)
1. School discipline. 2. Classroom management. 3. Restraint of patients. 4. Self-control. I. Kentley, Laura E.
LB3012.2.T565 2009
371.5'4--dc22

2010012291

Published by Nova Science Publishers, Inc. ✦ New York

Contents

PREFACE

This book explores the utilization of seclusions and restraints in schools. In certain circumstances, teachers and other staff may decide that it is necessary to restrain or seclude children in order to protect them from harming themselves or others. Some doctors and teachers contend that using seclusions and restraints can reduce injury and agitation and that it would be very difficult for organizations to run programs for children and adults with special needs without being able to use these methods. The authors highlight cases where staff at some programs employed unsafe restraint techniques, resulting in the death and abuse of teens in their care. Recent reports by advocacy groups indicate that similar restraint techniques have been used at public and private schools throughout the country.

Chapters 1 through 6 feature testimony before the U. S. House of Representatives.

Chapter 7 - GAO recently testified before the Committee regarding allegations of death and abuse at residential programs for troubled teens. Recent reports indicate that vulnerable children are being abused in other settings. For example, one report on the use of restraints and seclusions in schools documented cases where students were pinned to the floor for hours at a time, handcuffed, locked in closets, and subjected to other acts of violence. In some of these cases, this type of abuse resulted in death.

Given these reports, the Committee asked GAO to (1) provide an overview of seclusions and restraint laws applicable to children in public and private schools, (2) verify whether allegations of student death and abuse from the use of these methods are widespread, and (3) examine the facts and circumstances surrounding cases where a student died or suffered abuse as a result of being secluded or restrained.

GAO reviewed federal and state laws and abuse allegations from advocacy groups, parents, and the media from the past two decades. GAO did not evaluate whether using restraints and seclusions can be beneficial. GAO examined documents related to closed cases, including police and autopsy reports and school policies. GAO also interviewed parents, attorneys, and school officials and conducted searches to determine the current employment status of staff involved in the cases.

Chapter 8 - Seclusion and restraint have been used in various situations to deal with violent or noncompliant behavior. Because of recent congressional interest in the use of seclusion and restraint in schools, this report focuses on the legal issues concerning the use of these techniques in schools, including their application both to children covered by the Individuals with Disabilities Education Act (IDEA) and to those not covered by IDEA.

Several recent reports have documented instances of deaths and injuries resulting from the use of seclusion or restraints in schools, but there is no general reporting requirement so the exact parameters of the problem are unknown. On May 19, 2009, in conjunction with a hearing by the House Education and Labor Committee, the Government Accountability Office (GAO) released a study examining the use of seclusion and restraint in the education setting, finding hundreds of cases of alleged abuse and death due to the use of seclusion and restraint. On July 31, 2009, the Secretary of Education sent letters to Chief State School Officers noting the problems identified by the GAO report and in the May 19 congressional hearing, encouraging each state to review its current policies, and stating that the Chief State School Officers would be contacted by the Department of Education (ED) by August 15, 2009, to discuss relevant state laws, regulations, policies, and guidance. The results of these discussions are to be posted on ED's website.

Federal law does not contain general provisions relating to the use of seclusion and restraints, and there are no specific federal laws concerning the use of seclusion and restraint in public schools. The Individuals with Disabilities Education Act requires a free appropriate public education for children with disabilities, and an argument could be made that some uses of seclusion and restraint would violate this requirement. In addition, certain procedures may violate constitutional rights or state laws. Although there are some judicial cases, they do not provide clear guidance on when, if ever, seclusion and restraint may be used in schools.

In: Time Out: Examining Seclusion and... ISBN: 978-1-60876-932-2
Editor: Laura E. Kentley

Chapter 1

EXAMINING THE ABUSIVE AND DEADLY USE OF SECLUSION AND RESTRAINT IN SCHOOLS

Ann Gaydos

Chairman Miller, other distinguished members of the House Education and Labor Committee, thank you for the opportunity to testify this morning on the issue of restraint and seclusion in schools. I am here today to discuss the story of what happened to my daughter Paige in the hope that my telling this story will eventually lead to a world where no other child has to suffer the same trauma she did.

Paige is our oldest child, and from a very young age had an intense interest in learning everything she could. At the age of eighteen months, she enjoyed working on jigsaw puzzles and could read off any car license plate. By two, she could recognize and draw any state in the United States. As she got older, she became interested in science, especially astronomy and geology. Paige was a self-confident, happy, energetic little girl who would start a project and remain enthusiastically focused on it until it was complete. As I said, Paige loved to learn and was like a sponge soaking up all the information she could get on a topic.

In the beginning of 2001, when she was seven years old, we became concerned about Paige's unusual intensity, and emotional and sensory sensitivities. Loud noises caused her acute pain and she quickly became overwhelmed and sometimes withdrawn in group situations. She did not always understand how to communicate appropriately. As a result, we had her evaluated. While she remained a cheerful, bubbly, hyper-focused little girl, she was tentatively diagnosed with bipolar disorder, a diagnosis that was later discarded, and with Asperger's Syndrome.

This came as an enormous shock to my husband and me, but we vowed to ensure that Paige would continue her education in an environment that allowed her to thrive. At the time we lived in California in a well respected school district and felt that our local schools could provide her an excellent education and some help with the complexities of social interaction. We contacted our school district to discuss where to send Paige, and eventually went to observe a classroom and talk to a teacher about having Paige attend that school.

Although Paige's diagnoses at the time had been discussed, the school conducted only a cursory Individualized Education Plan (IEP) and at no time was a behavioral plan for Paige ever devised. After observing the room and placing our trust in a teacher who claimed she could educate and help Paige, Paige started school that March in a mixed grade classroom--kindergarten through third grade.

Paige was then very small – barely 40 pounds. Within a week at her new school, she came home bruised and told me, "Mommy, my teacher hurt me and I couldn't breathe." Concerned about this occurrence, my husband went in the next day to speak to the teacher. The teacher stated that she could not have caused the bruise, but informed him that she had restrained Paige for refusing to stop wiggling a loose tooth while in time out by holding her. She explained that children were supposed to be bored in the time out cubicle and weren't allowed to play with anything, not even a loose tooth.

We were shocked that we had not been informed by the school of this use of force that had injured our daughter, and that such force could so easily be used for something as small as playing with a loose tooth in time out. At no time before Paige had stated was there a discussion about using restraints on her, but following the meeting we still felt inclined to trust and believe this teacher who had said she could help our daughter.

In June of 2001 my husband ran into a former aide from Paige's classroom who warned him that the teacher had lied to him about the tooth-wiggling incident and the resulting restraint. The aide said the teacher had not just held Paige, but had forced Paige face-down on the floor and sat on her. She told us that she had been concerned that the teacher was abusing children in the classroom and she had tried to raise her concerns with the teacher's actions first with her superiors, and then school district officials. However, no action was ever taken by the school or the school district on her concerns. In fact, the aide's attempt to expose a pattern of abuse by this teacher ultimately caused her to resign after the school declined to take any action against the teacher.

Following these revelations, we immediately asked for, and had, a meeting with the teacher and the principal to discuss what had happened to my daughter. However, the principal continued to unconditionally support the teacher. While my husband and I debated taking Paige out of the school, we did reach an agreement that Paige would no longer be restrained and I offered to come to the school to help should any crisis develop. With this agreement, we decided to allow Paige to remain at the school. However, while the restraints stopped for a little while, Paige continued to be subjected to lengthy time outs, in some cases over three hours.

The beginning of the new school year started out fine until November of 2001. At that time, Paige was hurt on two successive days after interactions with her teacher. The second injury was fairly serious – a severe bruise to the bridge of Paige's nose that lasted a week. Paige said that she had been roughly jerked off a chair for refusing to stand up, which caused her to hit her nose on the desk.

Given that we had an agreement to be contacted if a crisis should develop we were worried, and tried to contact the principal. However, we were not able to speak with the principal until a week after the event. At this time it was finally suggested that we should have an IEP meeting, but given the schedule it couldn't be until about a month later. My husband and I looked for an alternative placement for our daughter, but nothing suitable was then available.

At this IEP meeting, held in December of 2001, my husband and I were quite vociferous in insisting that Paige could not be restrained and that our daughter should not again be hurt or bruised by the teacher absent an emergency situation. We also expressed concern about the excessive time she was spending in time out and shared our belief that our daughter, like many anxious children, needed a supportive and soothing environment. Again, the teacher agreed to our suggestion that we be called immediately to collect Paige if she was having problems. For a short time, the IEP meeting helped to change the classroom environment from one that was aggressively punitive to one that was much more therapeutic and humane.

There followed a relatively good period of several months, punctuated by one incident. The teacher called me to collect Paige in April of 2002. She explained that Paige had refused to eat and so she had snatched Paige's burrito and smeared some of it in her hair. At trial, as Paige testified, we heard for the very first time that Paige felt she herself had been responsible for the incident. She said she blamed herself that so much food was smeared on her because she had "struggled." When asked why she had struggled, she said it was because she couldn't breathe as the teacher had tried to shove the burrito into her mouth and covered her nose and mouth.

That summer we decided to have Paige do summer school. Because of how our school system handles summer school, Paige had the same teacher for summer school that she had for the regular school year. In July of 2002, I was called to fetch Paige from school. The principal was very evasive, but eventually told me Paige had tried to run away from school. When I collected Paige, she seemed completely overwhelmed. She was in the school office with the teacher, the behaviorist, and the program therapist. They were all behaving strangely and nobody would look me in the face. Nobody mentioned that Paige had been restrained or hurt.

As we were driving home, Paige burst into tears and told me, "Mommy, I've been hurt all day." She showed me a severe abrasion on her upper right arm. However, she did not volunteer any information about the blow to her head until that evening. At that time, my husband noticed that she had a large bump on the upper right hand side of her head. I still did not know the full extent of this event, but I called the principal and said that Paige would not be returning to summer school and told her how upset I was that nobody told me anything about what had happened. During this call, the principal informed me Paige had been given an ice pack to the head, but nothing more about the incident.

Paige's version of this culminating incident has never wavered and is entirely consistent with the nature and location of her injuries. Paige arrived at school that morning and saw the teacher on the way from the bus into the school. Something in the teacher's demeanor that day absolutely frightened Paige and she decided it was safer to try and walk home than go to school that day. As she started to walk home, an aide stopped her and was able to bring Paige to the classroom without the use of a restraint. However, even though we had an agreement to contact me or my husband, we did not get a call from the school and the situation continued to escalate even though Paige was not a threat to harm herself or others.

As the situation began to escalate, Paige was becoming increasingly agitated, her teacher took her into an empty classroom and grabbed Paige's wrists in her left hand and forced them up between Paige's shoulder blades. The teacher then grabbed Paige's left ankle in her right hand, lifted her off the ground, and drove her head-first into the ground at a slight angle to the vertical, causing her to land on the upper right side of her body so that she struck her head and shoulder. Not being informed of the trauma to her head when I picked her up could have had some serious long-term health consequences. We should have been watching Paige for possible signs of a concussion that afternoon and any possible subdural hemorrhage.

As fate would have it, the following day Paige had an appointment with her neuropsychologist at Stanford. Paige's neuropsychologist noticed the abrasion on Paige's arm and the palpable bump on her head and questioned her about where it had occurred. She then called me in and told me she felt Paige had been abused and that she had to report the incident to Child Protective Services (CPS).

Unfortunately, CPS had no jurisdiction over public school teachers and referred the matter to the police who came to our house that evening. They photographed Paige's arm, but the case was not ultimately prosecuted. We were given many reasons for this decision, which included the police's confidence that the situation would be handled internally by the school administration and board.

However, the faith of the police in the school administration or school board was misplaced in Paige's situation. We complained to the administration and wrote to the school board. Only one board member ever responded, and his advice was to sue the district. Nobody from the district ever called to ask how Paige was doing or suggested helping her in any way. We also could get no explanation out of anybody as to what had really happened to her.

No documentation or emergency intervention reports were ever filed for any of the incidents, despite the fact that this school district had been censured for absence of documentation following a complaint to the state about the same teacher four years previously.

Given our desire for Paige to receive a quality education and the distrust we had for that to occur at her old school, we decided to place Paige in a private school for special needs children, the Children's Health Council (CHC). However, because the school district failed to meet their requirement to pay for Paige's education at CHC, Paige missed eight months of school until that matter was resolved.

Once Paige began at CHC we met another child that had suffered great trauma at the hands of Paige's old teacher. This student had been in Paige's old classroom one year before Paige had started at the school and ultimately ended up at CHC because of the abuse he had received. This little boy was kept in a seclusion time out for the entire school day (8:30 a.m. to 2:35 p.m.) for 19 successive school days. He was also denied food, water, and bathroom access during this time. In addition, he came home with unexplained injuries which lead to his mother withdrawing the boy and sending him to CHC. We also learned that the mother had complained to CPS and the police about these incidents and a police report had been filed in this case.

We were horrified that this was at least the second instance of a CPS and police report being filed about the same teacher, and we as parents of a potential student of this teacher had not been informed of this before sending Paige to that school! On learning about this similar situation, we again wrote letters to the school board and the school superintendent. Finally, after again receiving no response to these letters, and being told that CPS and the police could not help, we decided to take the advice of the school board member that had said we should sue the school district, which we did in 2003. It was through this lawsuit that we learned of many other complaints against the teacher which we as parents (along with the many other families that had sent their children to this school) had not been informed about before sending our children to the school.

The trial had the absurdity of a Monty Python sketch about it as the story they tried to portray kept changing, and the school district attacked everyone other than the real perpetrators. One of the arguments that the district attempted to make was that our motive was to enrich ourselves through this lawsuit. Let me assure you that nothing could be further from the truth. We had offered to settle the lawsuit prior to trial for the costs of our legal fees, but we made it absolutely clear that we would not accept a confidentiality clause. After having met the other child at CHC that had been abused by the same teacher and learning of other stories through the lawsuit, we could not allow this to be swept under the rug through the use of a confidentiality clause.

Ultimately the jurors were unanimous in their verdict and found the teacher, principal, and district liable for damages. These damages are in a trust fund for Paige which she can access when she turns 18. Having to get the school district to recognize the problems with this teacher through a lawsuit was the last way in the world that this should have been addressed. It would have been much easier, and safer for many children, if the school district had taken seriously the allegations of abuse and neglect against this teacher at an earlier time, or if the school board had chosen to address the problem later.

We wish this was like the fairy tale stories we used to read to Paige as a little girl where you say, "and everyone lived happily ever after." Unfortunately, this is not the case. After we had withdrawn Paige from her old school, the teacher returned to the classroom as though nothing had happened. Shortly thereafter, a program therapist had occasion to call Child Protective Services after the teacher threatened a child with a pair of scissors. As was mentioned earlier, CPS has no jurisdiction over public school teachers and suggested to the therapist that she should call the police or speak to the administration. She spoke to the administration and the teacher finally left the school.

However, while she may have left that school, she went to work for another school district in California shortly thereafter. Since there was no central database established or requirement for schools to check for police or CPS reports, the school district did not know about these past incidents. To this day, the teacher still holds a valid California teaching license.

Paige is now 15, and has never fully recovered from these experiences. While still very intelligent, Paige has lost the enthusiasm she used to have for learning. She has since never achieved academically at the stellar level she did before these experiences. She is still afraid of schools, but she no longer hides beneath the desk as she used to do at her old school and at CHC when she first started there. We also believe that the events that occurred in this classroom kept her from being properly diagnosed for years delaying the ability to get her the proper services and supports.

We love our daughter with all our heart, and believe she will achieve great things in her life, but we are saddened by the tremendous loss of innocence and potential that she suffered at the hands of that teacher and the entire school administration that ignored these events. We tremble when we hear the stories from other parents about the long-term consequences that their children suffered from the same school system.

If we could go back and change history for our daughter we would. We unfortunately cannot do that, but hope that my being here to convey Paige's story along with the other witnesses testifying today will eventually lead to a world where thc things that happened to Paige will no longer happen again.

Again, thank you for the opportunity to testify today.

In: Time Out: Examining Seclusion and... ISBN: 978-1-60876-932-2
Editor: Laura E. Kentley

Chapter 2

TESTIMONY BEFORE THE HOUSE EDUCATION AND LABOR COMMITTEE

Elizabeth Hanselman

Mr. Chairman and Members of the Committee:

Thank you for the opportunity to speak to you on this important topic.

In 2001, Illinois enacted legislation (P.A. 91-600) to specifically address the issues of seclusion (known as "isolated time out" in IL) and physical restraint in public schools. The Illinois State Board of Education, in collaboration with stakeholders around the State, developed rules governing the use of isolated time out and physical restraint. We relied upon information from research and evidence-based practices. We also reviewed information from other State agencies and a couple of other states with existing rules. Illinois' rules became effective in January of 2002. Those rules:

- Apply to all students in Illinois, not only those with disabilities
- Limit the employment of isolated time out and physical restraint to be used only to preserve the safety of self or others, and
- Prohibit the use of seclusion or restraint for the purpose of punishment or exclusion

In the case of isolated time out, Illinois rules

- Impose time limits, and
- Require continuing visual monitoring of and communication with the student

In the case of physical restraint, Illinois rules only allow the use of physical restraint when

- The student poses a physical risk to self or others
- There is no medical contraindication to its use, and
- Staff applying the restraint have been trained in safe application in accordance with the rules, within the past 2 years, as indicated by written evidence

Further restrictions on the use of physical restraint include

- Time limits
- Prohibiting the use of chemical or mechanical restraints, and
- Requiring that students who communicate via sign language or augmentative devices be allowed to have their hands free of restraint

Our rules further require

- Specific documentation of each incident of seclusion or restraint
- Written notification to parents or guardians within 24 hours, and
- Review of, or development of, the student's individual behavioral intervention plan

Seclusion and restraint procedures should only be implemented as safety measures. The need for seclusion and restraint is in part the result of insufficient knowledge, skills and systems of prevention and behavior support. The majority of behaviors which result in the use of seclusion or restraint can be prevented by early identification and intensive interventions – implemented within a school- wide system of behavioral support.

For the past ten years, the Illinois State Board of Education has invested in the implementation of School-wide Positive Behavior and Intervention Supports (PBIS). PBIS is a systems approach to establishing the social culture needed for schools to achieve social and academic gains while minimizing problem behavior for all students. PBIS is not a curriculum, but rather a framework for decision making that guides the implementation of evidence-based academic and behavioral practices. Key to the implementation of PBIS is the recognition that we must teach and acknowledge behavioral and social skills, just as we teach academic skills. School-wide PBIS emphasizes:

- The implementation of evidence-based practices,
- School, district and state systems that support the implementation of these practices, and
- Ongoing collection and use of data for decision-making.

Drs. Robert Horner and George Sugai of the National PBIS Center note that these elements are operationalized by five guiding principles:

- Invest first in prevention to establish a foundation intervention that is empirically validated to be effective, efficient and sustainable.
- Teach and acknowledge appropriate behavior before relying on negative consequences.
- Use regular "universal screening" to identify students who need more intense support and provide that support as early as possible, and with the intensity needed to meet the student's need.
- Establish a continuum of behavioral and academic interventions for use when students are identified as needing more intense support.
- Use progress monitoring to assess (a) the fidelity with which support is provided and (b) the impact of support on student academic and social outcomes. Use data for continuous improvement of support.

Over 1,000 schools in Illinois now implement PBIS as part of a statewide network under the direction of Dr. Lucille Eber. This includes elementary schools, middle schools, high schools, alternative schools, residential schools and even juvenile correction centers. Data collection over these past 10 years shows significant reductions in office disciplinary referrals, suspensions and expulsions – resulting in increased time for academic instruction and learning. Staff and students alike at schools that implement PBIS experience improved measures of school safety. And, in Illinois, schools that implement PBIS with fidelity show improved academic outcomes as measured by our Illinois Standards Achievement Test.

Illinois schools which have achieved full implementation of PBIS also show greater capacity to support students with the most complex emotional/behavioral needs. Data indicates that these schools have a reduction in the number of instances which require intensive interventions (including seclusion and restraint), increased effectiveness of individual behavior support plans, and improvement in the maintenance of behavior support gains achieved through these individual support plans.

Illinois data shows that implementation of school-wide PBIS can have a positive impact in all programs, including:

- Reduction of the use of restraint in a separate facility for students with emotional disorders by more than 50% in the first year of implementing PBIS
- Reduction in the occurrence of critical incidents by more than 60% following implementation in a youth correctional center

Illinois is now working with the National Scaling Up effort to build the statewide infrastructure to support the expansion of integrated evidence-based practices – which includes PBIS - to every one of the more than 4,100 schools in our state.

Illinois is committed to supporting not only the academic, but also the social and emotional development of all students. To that end, Illinois became the first state to establish Social and Emotional Learning Standards in 2004. We continue to support training and technical assistance to schools in the effective implementation of those standards.

Based on our experience in Illinois, we urge the adoption of a national model policy on the use of seclusion and restraint. This can only be effective when coupled with a strong commitment and investment in the training and ongoing support of staff in the use of evidence-based prevention strategies.

Respectfully submitted,
Elizabeth Hanselman
Director of Special Education
Illinois State Board of Education

SUBTITLE A. SUBCHAPTER A

Section 1.285 Requirements for the Use of Isolated Time Out and Physical Restraint

Isolated time out and physical restraint as defined in this Section shall be used only as means of maintaining discipline in schools (that is, as means of maintaining a safe and orderly environment for learning) and only to the extent that they are necessary to preserve the safety of students and others. Neither isolated time out nor physical restraint shall be used in administering discipline to individual students, i.e., as a form of punishment. Nothing in this Section or in Section 1.280 of this Part shall be construed as regulating the restriction of students' movement when that restriction is for a purpose other than the maintenance of an orderly environment (e.g., the appropriate use of safety belts in vehicles).

(a) "Isolated time out" means the confinement of a student in a time-out room or some other enclosure, whether within or outside the classroom, from which the student's egress is restricted. The use of isolated time out shall be subject to the following requirements.

(1) Any enclosure used for isolated time out shall:

(A) have the same ceiling height as the surrounding room or rooms and be large enough to accommodate not only the student being isolated but also any other individual who is required to accompany that student;

(B) be constructed of materials that cannot be used by students to harm themselves or others, be free of electrical outlets, exposed wiring, and other objects that could be used by students to harm themselves or others, and be designed so that students cannot climb up the walls (including walls far enough apart so as not to offer the student being isolated sufficient leverage for climbing); and

(C) be designed to permit continuous visual monitoring of and communication with the student.

(2) If an enclosure used for isolated time out is fitted with a door, either a steel door or a wooden door of solid-core construction shall be used. If the door includes a viewing panel, the panel shall be unbreakable.

(3) An adult who is responsible for supervising the student shall remain within two feet of the enclosure.

(4) The adult responsible for supervising the student must be able to see the student at all times. If a locking mechanism is used on the enclosure, the mechanism shall be constructed so that it will engage only when a key, handle, knob, or other similar device is being held in position by a person, unless the mechanism is an electrically or electronically controlled one that is automatically released when the building's fire alarm system is triggered. Upon release of the locking mechanism by the supervising adult, the door must be able to be opened readily.

(b) "Physical restraint" means holding a student or otherwise restricting his or her movements. "Physical restraint" as permitted pursuant to this Section includes only the use of specific, planned techniques (e.g., the "basket hold" and "team control").

(c) The requirements set forth in subsections (d) through (h) of this Section shall not apply to the actions described in this subsection (c) because, pursuant to Section 10-20.33 of the School Code [105 ILCS 5/10-20.33], "RESTRAINT" DOES NOT INCLUDE MOMENTARY PERIODS OF PHYSICAL RESTRICTION BY DIRECT PERSON-TO-PERSON CONTACT, WITHOUT THE AID OF MATERIAL OR MECHANICAL DEVICES, ACCOMPLISHED WITH LIMITED FORCE AND DESIGNED TO:

(1) PREVENT A STUDENT FROM COMPLETING AN ACT THAT WOULD RESULT IN POTENTIAL PHYSICAL HARM TO HIMSELF, HERSELF, OR ANOTHER OR DAMAGE TO PROPERTY; OR

(2) REMOVE A DISRUPTIVE STUDENT WHO IS UNWILLING TO LEAVE THE AREA VOLUNTARILY.

(d) The use of physical restraint shall be subject to the following requirements.

(1) Pursuant to Section 10-20.33 of the School Code, physical restraint may only be employed when:

(A) THE STUDENT POSES A PHYSICAL RISK TO HIMSELF, HERSELF, OR OTHERS,

(B) THERE IS NO MEDICAL CONTRAINDICATION TO ITS USE, AND

(C) THE STAFF APPLYING THE RESTRAINT HAVE BEEN TRAINED IN ITS SAFE APPLICATION as specified in subsection (h) (2) of this Section.

(2) Students shall not be subjected to physical restraint for using profanity or other verbal displays of disrespect for themselves or others. A verbal threat shall not be considered as constituting a physical danger unless a student also demonstrates a means of or intent to carry out the threat.

(3) Except as permitted by the administrative rules of another State agency operating or licensing a facility in which elementary or secondary educational services are provided (e.g., the Illinois Department of Corrections or the Illinois Department of Human Services), mechanical or chemical restraint (i.e., the use of any device other than personal physical force to restrict the limbs, head, or body) shall not be employed.

(4) Medically prescribed restraint procedures employed for the treatment of a physical disorder or for the immobilization of a person in connection with a medical or surgical procedure shall not be used as means of physical restraint for purposes of maintaining discipline.

(5) Any application of physical restraint shall take into consideration the safety and security of the student. Further, physical restraint shall not rely upon pain as an intentional method of control.

(6) In determining whether a student who is being physically restrained should be removed from the area where such restraint was initiated, the supervising adult(s) shall consider the potential for injury to the student, the student's need for privacy, and the educational and emotional well-being of other students in the vicinity.

(7) If physical restraint is imposed upon a student whose primary mode of communication is sign language or an augmentative mode, the student shall be permitted to have his or her hands free of restraint for brief periods, unless the supervising adult determines that such freedom appears likely to result in harm to the student or others.

(e) Time Limits

(1) A student shall not be kept in isolated time out for more than 30 minutes after he or she ceases presenting the specific behavior for which isolated time out was imposed or any other behavior for which it would be an appropriate intervention.

(2) A student shall be released from physical restraint immediately upon a determination by the staff member administering the restraint that the student is no longer in imminent danger of causing physical harm to himself, herself, or others.

(f) Documentation and Evaluation

(1) A written record of each episode of isolated time out or physical restraint shall be maintained in the student's temporary record. The official designated pursuant to Section 1.280(c) (3) of this Part shall also maintain a copy of each such record. Each such record shall include:

(A) the student's name;
(B) the date of the incident;
(C) the beginning and ending times of the incident;
(D) a description of any relevant events leading up to the incident;
(E) a description of any interventions used prior to the implementation of isolated time out or physical restraint;
(F) a description of the incident and/or student behavior that resulted in isolated time out or physical restraint;
(G) a log of the student's behavior in isolated time out or during physical restraint, including a description of the restraint technique(s) used and any other interaction between the student and staff;
(H) a description of any injuries (whether to students, staff, or others) or property damage;
(I) a description of any planned approach to dealing with the student's behavior in the future;
(J) a list of the school personnel who participated in the implementation, monitoring, and supervision of isolated time out or physical restraint;
(K) the date on which parental notification took place as required by subsection (g) of this Section.

(2) The school official designated pursuant to Section 1.280(c) (3) of this Part shall be notified of the incident as soon as

possible, but no later than the end of the school day on which it occurred.

(3) The record described in subsection (f) (1) of this Section shall be completed by the beginning of the school day following the episode of isolated time out or physical restraint.

(4) The requirements of this subsection (f) (4) shall apply whenever an episode of isolated time out exceeds 30 minutes, an episode of physical restraint exceeds 15 minutes, or repeated episodes have occurred during any three-hour period.

(A) A certified staff person knowledgeable about the use of isolated time out or trained in the use of physical restraint, as applicable, shall evaluate the situation.

(B) The evaluation shall consider the appropriateness of continuing the procedure in use, including the student's potential need for medication, nourishment, or use of a restroom, and the need for alternate strategies (e.g., assessment by a mental health crisis team, assistance from police, or transportation by ambulance).

(C) The results of the evaluation shall be committed to writing and copies of this documentation shall be placed into the student's temporary student record and provided to the official designated pursuant to Section 1.280(c) (3) of this Part.

(5) When a student has first experienced three instances of isolated time out or physical restraint, the school personnel who initiated, monitored, and supervised the incidents shall initiate a review of the effectiveness of the procedure(s) used and prepare an individual behavior plan for the student that provides either for continued use of these interventions or for the use of other, specified interventions. The plan shall be placed into the student's temporary student record. The review shall also consider the student's potential need for an alternative program or for special education.

(A) The district or other entity serving the student shall invite the student's parent(s) or guardian(s) to participate in this review and shall provide ten days' notice of its date, time, and location.

(B) The notification shall inform the parent(s) or guardian(s) that the student's potential need for special education or an alternative program will be considered and that the results of the review will be entered into the temporary student record.

(g) Notification to Parents

(1) A district whose policies on the maintenance of discipline include the use of isolated time out or physical restraint shall notify parents to this effect as part of the information distributed annually or upon enrollment pursuant to Sections 10-20.14 and 14-8.05(c) of the School Code [105 ILCS 5/10-20.14 and 14-8.05(c)].

(2) Within 24 hours after any use of isolated time out or physical restraint, the school district or other entity serving the student shall send written notice of the incident to the student's parent(s), unless the parent has provided the district or other entity with a written waiver of this requirement for notification. Such notification shall include the student's name, the date of the incident, a description of the intervention used, and the name of a contact person with a telephone number to be called for further information.

(h) Requirements for Training

(1) Isolated Time Out
Each district, cooperative, or joint agreement whose policy permits the use of isolated time out shall provide orientation to its staff members covering at least the written procedure established pursuant to Section 1.280(c) (2) of this Part.

(2) Physical Restraint

(A) Physical restraint as defined in this Section shall be applied only by individuals who have received systematic training that includes all the elements described in subsection (h) (2) (B) of this Section and who have received a certificate of completion or other written evidence of participation. An individual who applies physical restraint shall use only techniques in which he or she has received such training within the preceding two years, as indicated by written evidence of participation.

(B) Training with respect to physical restraint may be provided either by the employer or by an external entity and shall include, but need not be limited to:

(i) appropriate procedures for preventing the need for physical restraint, including the de-escalation of problematic behavior, relationship-building, and the use of alternatives to restraint;

(ii) a description and identification of dangerous behaviors on the part of students that may indicate the need for physical restraint and methods for evaluating the risk of harm in individual situations in order to determine whether the use of restraint is warranted;

(iii) the simulated experience of administering and receiving a variety of physical restraint techniques, ranging from minimal physical involvement to very controlling interventions;

(iv) instruction regarding the effects of physical restraint on the person restrained, including instruction on monitoring physical signs of distress and obtaining medical assistance;

(v) instruction regarding documentation and reporting requirements and investigation of injuries and complaints; and

(vi) demonstration by participants of proficiency in administering physical restraint.

(C) An individual may provide training to others in a particular method of physical restraint only if he or she has received written evidence of completing training in that technique that meets the requirements of subsection (h) (2) (B) of this Section within the preceding one-year period.

(Source: Added at 26 Ill. Reg. 1157, effective January 16, 2002)

Chapter 3

EXAMINING THE ABUSIVE AND DEADLY USE OF SECLUSION AND RESTRAINT IN SCHOOLS

V. Mary Kealy

Chairman Miller, Ranking Member McKeon and Members of the Committee:

Thank you for inviting me to testify to you today regarding the use of "seclusion and restraint" from a public school administrator's perspective.

My name is Mary Kealy and I am the Assistant Superintendent for Pupil Services for Loudoun County Public Schools, a large growing and thriving school division of over 57,000 students in the Washington, DC metropolitan area. I speak to you from experience in my current role and from several years of experience in various administrative roles in New Jersey and Virginia, including principal of both public and private special education schools.

Among other areas, including guidance, psychology, social work, attendance and health services, my department provides oversight, direction and services for special education and related professional development to administrative, teaching and support staff in 75 schools, grades Pre-K through 12. Currently, about 6,000 of these students receive special education services.

It is apparent that this topic is of concern as we continue to strive for safe and orderly environments in our public schools. We must ensure that all children are treated with respect and dignity and that the learning environment is safe for all students and staff. We all know there is a high correlation between positive and safe school environments and student achievement.

Given the concern surrounding the issues related to this topic, I would like to offer comments on the following: the use of seclusion and restraint, the student population affected, prevention focus, staff development and training/best practices, implementation challenges, recommendations and some information about professional resources and advocacy efforts.

I will briefly address each of these areas.

USE OF SECLUSION AND RESTRAINT

I'd like to begin by emphasizing that neither the use of seclusion or restraint is considered a "best educational practice" and is not recommended as a typical educational strategy in our schools. In fact, the use of these practices is strongly discouraged and an emphasis on positive behavior supports is encouraged. *The American Association of School Administrators believes that monitored seclusion and restraints should be used as a last resort but must be an option for staff working with students who are out of control and pose a danger to themselves and others.* When there is a need to manage aggressive or violent behavior of students in emergency situations, there must be a balance between maintaining an effective and safe learning environment for children and school staff and safeguarding the rights and protections of students. However, their use may be considered as an option on the continuum of behavioral interventions as a safety measure of last resort, when all other interventions have been tried and the student may be a danger to himself or others. It is important for school divisions to ensure that any behavior management techniques used are appropriate. Physical restraint and seclusion should only be used in emergency situations, when other less intrusive alternatives have failed.

STUDENT POPULATIONS MOST AFFECTED

Special education students with emotional, behavioral or significant cognitive disabilities have historically been the students requiring the most intense behavioral interventions for aggressive and other challenging behaviors. Programs for students with emotional disabilities, autism and multiple disabilities are typically structured to provide the continuum of supports, services and resources to address severe behavioral issues. However, as we continue to meet the least restrictive environment requirements of the Individuals with Disabilities Education Act (IDEA), several of these students spend all or part of their day in general education environments. As a result, both general and special education staff need to receive the appropriate training and supports to address the needs of these special populations in inclusive environments. Therefore, an inclusive approach to prevention, training and support is recommended as best practice. However, it is essential that special education teachers of students with the most challenging behavior issues take a leadership role in implementing a team-based approach to address challenging behaviors as part of a schoolwide approach.

PREVENTION

Based on over 30 years of research, Drs. George Sugai and Rob Horner, co-directors of the US Department of Education, Centers for Positive Behavior Intervention and Support (www.pbis.org), support the use of schoolwide strategies as a proactive way to address behaviors in schools and promote success for all students., Using the 3-tiered approach, students are provided with a continuum of behavior supports based on their needs at each level: schoolwide (80%), targeted interventions for students requiring more specialized strategies (10-15%) and individualized(5- 10%). It is these students at the top tier who need the specialized interventions and alternatives required to meet their needs.

The appropriate use of physical restraint may be a tool, under certain circumstances, used as a last resort for students who exhibit out of control or dangerous behavior and may injure themselves or others. In order for physical restraint to be used effectively, it is essential that behavioral interventions which might prevent the need for restraint are in place. Included among them should be a variety of positive behavioral supports including establishing and teaching behavioral expectations, recognizing and reinforcing positive behavior, providing mental health services and interventions, and relying on functional behavior assessment and related intervention plans for any student whose behavior indicates a need for intervention. Without these, the number of "emergency" situations which might require restraint would be much greater than would otherwise be necessary. It is essential that behavioral interventions which might prevent the need for restraint are in place and staff have the resources and support to implement them.

Staff Development and Training

Although the research on best practice calls for a focus on prevention and the use of positive behavior supports and interventions, it is apparent that in specific emergency situations, the use of appropriate restraint as a tool may be necessary. If either seclusion or restraint are used in extreme or emergency situations, it is critical that anyone using these procedures be carefully trained in all aspects of their use. In addition to training in positive behavior supports, special education staff should receive mandatory training in behavioral techniques designed to de-escalate and resolve conflicts to avoid and defuse crisis situations. Conflict de-escalation appears to be a necessary intervention to prevent the use of restraint as well as useful in preventing and defusing behavior problems both for students with emotional or behavioral disorders as well as all students who may engage in power struggles or escalate emotional crises for other reasons.

In my experience with best practice models, the systematic training provided through the Mandt System (www.mandtsystem.com) provides educators with the necessary components of a comprehensive training program for school staff to be certified in these techniques. In my school division and others I have worked in, the basic level of training is mandated for special education teachers, while other more advanced levels involving more specific technical skills and intervention is required for teachers of students with severe cognitive challenges as well as students with autism and emotional disability. The appropriate use of physical restraint is taught at the advanced level. General education staff may register for components of the advanced training with the approval of their principal or supervisor, thus allowing then to learn techniques that will prevent injury to themselves or others.

Staff receives certification after successful course completion which must be renewed annually. It is important for school divisions to build the capacity to train staff annually, renew certifications and monitor staff implementation of these best practices to ensure appropriate implementation of these techniques and procedures. Resources must be provided to school divisions to allow for the successful implementation of the training and follow-up support required.

Implementation Challenges

There are several challenges that prevent the successful implementation of the proactive approaches for addressing effective use of appropriate behavioral interventions including the use of physical restraint and seclusion, when necessary. School divisions must provide the:

- administrative oversight for direction to schools and staff;
- policies, guidelines and procedures to ensure consistent and appropriate implementation;
- systems approach to behavioral intervention using best practices approaches;
- recurrent training to ensure annual updates and staff recertification;
- resources and support for school staff to participate in training;
- follow-up support by behavior specialists or other staff through consultation and support activities; and
- capacity-building training to sustain efforts over time.

Recommendations

The following recommendations or guiding principles are intended to frame any goals or policies of school divisions to diminish the need to use seclusion or restraint procedures in school settings.

- All children should receive necessary educational and mental health interventions and supports in a safe and least restrictive environment.
- School staff should receive training in the use of proactive, research–based strategies focused on preventive techniques, such as schoolwide positive behavior supports and interventions.
- A continuum of behavioral interventions and supports should be provided routinely to all children.
- All staff should participate in specialized training to include conflict de-escalation training and techniques to avoid and defuse crisis and conflict situations.
- Schools must have the necessary resources, staffing levels to provide positive supports to students and on-going training and support for

staff to sustain best practice interventions for students with challenging behaviors.

- In accordance with IDEA, students exhibiting a pattern of behavior impeding their learning or that of others should receive a functional behavior assessment and related behavior intervention plan which incorporates positive behavioral interventions, including instruction in appropriate behavior and strategies to deescalate their own behavior.
- The US Department of Education should provide more research on the use of seclusion and restraint in the school setting in at least four different settings, primary grades, upper elementary grades, middle schools and high schools. Students at each level are so different that research must identify age appropriate interventions to avoid the use of seclusion and restraint and how as a last resort such methods can be used most effectively for the progress of students and safety of the student, other students and staff, and volunteers.

Professional Resources and Advocacy Efforts

Many states provide guidelines or for the development of policies and procedures and to assist school divisions and public school programs that will help in situations involving the management of challenging student behavior with reference to the state code and regulations.

For example, the Virginia Department of Education has provided such a document for school divisions: **Guidelines for the Development of Policies and Procedures for Managing Student Behaviors in Emergency Situations in Virginia Public Schools- Focusing on Physical Restraint and Seclusion, November 2005. (www.doe.virginia.gov/VDOE/sess/)**

Additionally, the Council of Children with Behavior Disorders, a division of the Council for Exceptional Children (CEC), has done extensive work on developing comprehensive position documents on both **Seclusion and Physical Restraint Procedures in School Settings**. The draft documents represent research and best practices from the field coordinated by Dr. Reece Peterson, University of Nebraska-Lincoln, Lincoln, NE and Dr. Susan Albrecht, Ball State University, Muncie, IN. They are currently being vetted to other CEC divisions, such as the Council of Administrators of Special Education (CASE), for review and comments. As President-Elect of CASE, I am currently involved in this review. Upon completion, I am hopeful that this important work will inform the practice of those administrators and teachers working in school settings and present clear policy recommendations and best practices with prevention as the primary focus.

I thank you again for the opportunity to speak with you today and share some insights into the local school division perspective on this issue. I hope that we can work together to ensure safe, positive learning environments for all students in our schools. I look forward to answering your questions.

In: Time Out: Examining Seclusion and... ISBN: 978-1-60876-932-2
Editor: Laura E. Kentley

Chapter 4

STATEMENT OF CONGRESSMAN GEORGE MILLER, CHAIRMAN, EDUCATION & LABOR COMMITTEE*

United States House of Representatives

CHAIRMAN MILLER STATEMENT AT COMMITTEE HEARING ON "EXAMINING THE ABUSIVE AND DEADLY USE OF SECLUSION AND RESTRAINT IN SCHOOLS"

Washington, D.C. – *Below are the prepared remarks of U.S. Rep. George Miller (D- CA), chairman of the House Education and Labor Committee, for a committee hearing on "Examining the Abusive and Deadly Use of Seclusion and Restraint in Schools."*

Today's hearing is the first ever Congressional investigation of the abusive and deadly misuse of seclusion and restraint in our schools.

Unfortunately, the issue of abuse and seclusion and restraint of children is not new to this committee.

Last year, we held hearings to examine allegations of abuse and death of teens in residential treatment programs, which led us to pass H.R. 911 earlier this year.

---

* This is an edited, reformatted and augmented version of a U. S. House of Representatives publication dated May 2009.

This bill establishes basic health and safety standards in those programs and was passed with overwhelming bipartisan support.

That's because when we're talking about keeping our children safe, it isn't a partisan issue – it's a moral obligation.

Sadly, we're here again to talk about seclusion and restraint. But this time, we're looking at children in our nation's public and private schools.

In January, I asked the Government Accountability Office to investigate whether allegations of deadly and abusive seclusion and restraint in the schools are founded and widespread.

Simply put, the answer is yes.

What they found is alarming, eye opening and it is going to send shockwaves into every corner of this country. And it should.

The GAO will tell us very shortly that hundreds of students in this country have been victims of abuse in school.

In some cases, this abuse has been fatal.

Though it is not limited to students with disabilities, it is happening more often to these vulnerable children.

We will hear today from two parents, Ann Gaydos and Toni Price, whose lives have been devastated by teachers and classroom aides who went too far.

I thank them for traveling here today and for having the courage to speak publicly about the trauma they have experienced.

Federal law restricts the use of seclusion and restraint to emergency circumstances for children in hospitals, community-based residential treatment facilities, and other facilities supported by federal dollars.

Yet these rules do not apply to public or private schools.

This means an untrained medical professional is forbidden to inappropriately restrain a patient; and if they do, there are laws specifically targeted to address such behavior.

But untrained classroom staffs are abusing students in schools without any accountability because of a lack of federal oversight. Our children are bearing the physical and emotional burden of a system designed to fail them.

State regulation and oversight varies greatly; many states have no laws specifically governing the appropriate use of seclusion and restraint in schools.

And, parents are often unaware of the use of these abuses – until their child comes home with bruises or, tragically, can't come home at all.

School is a place for students to learn, grow and thrive. Families and communities trust teachers and school administrators to keep children safe.

Yet some educators are misusing behavioral interventions – interventions that were intended only to be used in emergencies as a last resort – for discipline or convenience in non-emergency situations.

Last year alone, in my home state of California, districts reported more than 14,300 cases of seclusion, restraint and other "emergency" interventions. We don't know how many of these cases were real emergencies.

Recent news reports document appalling stories of teachers tying children to chairs, taping their mouths shut, using handcuffs, denying them food, fracturing bones, locking them in small dark spaces, and sitting on them until they turn blue.

One might start to wonder what could possibly cause a teacher or classroom aide to abuse a child this way.

Well, we know what these children did: they fidgeted in their chairs or they were unwilling to follow directions. In some cases, they left the room or avoided a difficult task.

These behaviors are often a manifestation of the child's disability, yet the teachers, who are too often not appropriately trained to physically intervene, are restraining children anyway.

The vast majority of teachers and staff working in the schools are caring professionals who on a daily basis are making a difference in the lives of the children they teach.

But the teachers and staff who are abusing children must be held accountable for their actions.

It is wholly unacceptable for the egregious abuse of a child to be considered less criminal because it happened in a classroom.

It should be the opposite.

At a minimum, we should ensure our teachers are supported appropriately through training and classroom management resources.

I know educators are struggling with managing student behavior on many levels. Bullying and school violence are difficult issues that must be addressed.

Teachers and staff need to feel safe themselves, which is exactly why we must support ways to reduce problem behaviors in schools.

Approaches such as School Wide Positive Behavior Support can help establish a social culture and positive environment that uses data-driven decision-making to foster appropriate behavior and improve academic achievement.

Such practices have been shown to reduce office discipline referrals and problematic behavior.

Children should not be abused in our classrooms under the guise of discipline or punishment.

This must stop now.

Families should never be left wondering whether their child is safe in the care of their school.

And teachers should not feel compelled to use "emergency" interventions to manage behavior on a regular basis.

Congress must step in and fill the void that has resulted in scars that may never heal for these children and their families who have been victims of this abuse. I hope the next step will be to enact a federal policy to ensure the tragic stories we will hear today will never occur again.

Thank you.

In: Time Out: Examining Seclusion and… ISBN: 978-1-60876-932-2
Editor: Laura E. Kentley

Chapter 5

TESTIMONY OF REECE L. PETERSON

L. Reece Peterson

Chairman Miller, Ranking member McKeon and Distinguished Committee members

My role is that of a researcher who along with other colleagues from around the country are attempting to understand the use of restraint and seclusion procedures in school settings. I have been a researcher and teacher educator in special education for more than 30 years. My purpose is to share with you what we know, or perhaps more accurately what we don't know about the use of restraint and seclusion in schools.

RESEARCH ON RESTRAINT AND SECLUSION

There is virtually no research about the number of situations which occur in schools where student behavior poses danger of physical injury to themselves, other students or staff. Similarly, there is no information about these situations are addressed- whether physical restraint (where an adult physically hold the student and prevents the student from moving) or seclusion procedures (where a student is placed in a special environment by themselves and prevented from leaving) – whether these were employed.

PURPOSE AND USE OF RESTRAINT AND SECLUSION

I believe that there is agreement among knowledgeable professional educators that physical restraint and seclusion procedures should only be used rarely in school settings to prevent injuries- when there is immediate danger of physical injury to someone- in "emergency situations." While some have suggested that both restraint and seclusion can be used to change student behavior, there is virtually no evidence to support their effectiveness for that purpose. (Seclusion should be distinguished from "time out from positive reinforcement" which does have evidence of potential value in changing behavior but which need not entail seclusion.) There is controversy regarding whether these procedures should also be employed when students may be causing serious damage to the school environment. Most would say that they should not be used in such situations because of the risks for injury from these procedures may be larger than the risks without such strategies.

Nevertheless there are some isolated studies and anecdotal evidence that these procedures are being used in a variety of other situations. In one study my colleagues and I found that the use of these procedures occurred for "student non-compliance", "leaving the learning environment", and other student behaviors which did not apparently entail danger of physical injury to anyone. [1] Similar instances of non-emergency use have occurred in many of the numerous news media reports.

According to anecdotal reports, these procedures have also been implemented inappropriately in other respects. Restraints have been conducted by people not trained to do so, without recognition of the physiological symptoms of distress such as restricted breathing, or they were conducted well past the time when the student has regained control. Seclusion has been employed in environments which are unsafe, without close monitoring of the student, and for extended (and inappropriate) lengths of time, etc. All of these situations defy commonly accepted professional guidelines for the use of these procedures.

How Many?

Since these reports are often the result of parent complaints or media reports, we do not know how many times these procedures are inappropriately employed with students. Yet there does appear to be a substantial number of these situations, and they appear to be scattered across the United States. It should be acknowledged that there may also be many situations across the US where these procedures are being used much more appropriately, and there may be little or no adverse affects because of their use in those situations.

State Policies

States have varied substantially in their supervision of these procedures in the schools. In recent studies my colleagues and I conducted we found that there are 21 states which have policies & 10 more with guidelines in place which address the use of physical restraint. Fourteen states reported no policies or guidelines.[2] For seclusion, there are about 17 states which have policies & 7 more with guidelines we could identify.[3] Most of the time both types of policies and guidelines were included in special education policies for those states, but all of these policies varied widely in their terminology, definitions, content.

Disability

It is important to note that the use of these procedures is not strictly an issue related to students with disabilities. While most of the instances of use of these procedures have apparently been for students with disabilities, some have not. School staff members who engage in restraint or seclusion may not be special education staff- - we currently do not know. Nor do we know their level of training on these topics.

RECOMMENDATIONS

There is concern among knowledgeable professionals regarding the deaths and injuries resulting from these procedures, concern that reasonable guidelines for their use are apparently not being followed, and concern for violation of human rights. Here are just a few key recommendations:

- Schools should focus on the *prevention* of behavior problems. To do that implementation of “Positive Behavior Supports”, and conflict de-escalation procedures may lessen the need for the use of restraint and seclusion procedures. Preventing the occurrence of dangerous student behavior should be a top priority.

- *Adequate staffing* in programs serving students where serious behavior issues could be reasonably predicted.

- *Appropriate and specific training* for staff members on these topics, tailored to the specific setting, students and behaviors.

- *A common framework* across states and schools which specifies the situations where these procedures could be appropriate, and where they are inappropriate and how they should be used.

- More consistent *emergency or safety planning* which involves parents and students when difficult behaviors can be anticipated. Improved communication with parents would be helpful.

- *Common debriefing and reporting procedures* to some outside of district agency, such as State Departments of Education, which is directed to provide *oversight*_and watch for excessive use of these procedures, and investigate and take corrective action where guidelines are not followed.

Currently a more comprehensive set of recommendations is being developed by the Council for Children with Behavior Disorders, a Division of the Council for Exceptional Children which address many of these issues. (See attachment #1 and related documents). Implementation of recommendations like these would be very helpful.

Respectfully,
Reece L. Peterson

ATTACHMENT#1 CCBD POSITION SUMMARY ON PHYSICAL RESTRAINT & SECLUSION PROCEDURES IN SCHOOL SETTINGS MAY 2009

This document is a summary of policy recommendations from two longer and more detailed documents available from the Council for Children with Behavioral Disorders (CCBD) regarding the use of physical restraint and seclusion procedures in schools.

Declaration of Principles

- CCBD supports the following principles as related to the use of restraint or seclusion procedures:
  - Behavioral interventions for children must promote the right of all children to be treated with dignity.
  - All children should receive necessary educational and mental health supports and programming in a safe and least-restrictive environment.
  - Positive and appropriate educational interventions, as well as mental health supports, should be provided routinely to all children who need them.
  - Behavioral interventions should emphasize prevention and creating positive behavioral supports.
  - Schools should have adequate staffing levels to effectively provide positive supports to student and should be staffed with appropriately trained personnel.
  - All staff in schools should have mandatory conflict de-escalation training, and conflict de-escalation techniques should be employed by all school staff to avoid and defuse crisis and conflict situations.
  - All children whose pattern of behavior impedes their learning or the learning of others should receive appropriate educational assessment, including Functional Behavioral Assessments followed by Behavioral Intervention Plans which incorporate appropriate positive behavioral interventions, including instruction in appropriate behavior and strategies to de-escalate their own behavior.

Recommendations

- CCBD believes that physical restraint or seclusion procedures should be used in school settings only when the physical safety of the student or others is in immediate danger.
- Mechanical or chemical restraints should never be used in school settings when their purpose is simply to manage or address student behavior (other than their use by law endorsement or when students in travel restraints in vehicles). Their use for other instructional related purposes should be supervised by qualified and trained individuals and in accord with professional standards for their use.
- Neither restraints nor seclusion should be used as a punishment to force compliance or as a substitute for appropriate educational support.
- CCBD calls for any school which employs physical restraint or seclusion procedures to have a written positive behavior support plan specific to that program, pre-established emergency procedures, specific procedures and training related to the use of restraint and seclusion, and data to support the implementation of the principles of positive behavior supports in that environment as well as data regarding the specific uses of restraint and seclusion.
- All seclusion environments should be safe and humane and should be inspected at least annually, not only by fire or safety inspectors but for programmatic implementation of guidelines and data related to its use.
- Any student in seclusion must be continuously observed by an adult both visually and aurally for the entire period of the seclusion. Occasional checks are not acceptable.
- CCBD calls for federal, state, and provincial legislation or regulation which would require the implementation of:
  - Recognition that restraint and seclusion procedures are emergency, not treatment, procedures.
  - Requirement that preventive measures such as conflict de-escalation procedures be in place in schools where restraints or seclusion will be employed.
  - Requirements that individualized safety plans are created for students whose behavior could reasonably be predicted to pose a danger. Those safety plans for students with disabilities must be created by the student's IEP team and included as a part of the

IEP. These plans can also be created for students without disabilities.
- Requirements that comprehensive debriefings occur after each use of restraint or seclusion and that reports of the incident are created
- Requirement that data on restraints and seclusion are reported to an outside agency such as the state or provincial department of education.

- CCBD does not believe that "guidelines" or "technical assistance documents" are generally adequate to regulate the use of these procedures since abuses continue to occur in states or provinces where guidelines are in place and these guidelines have few mechanisms for providing oversight or correction of abuses.
- CCBD calls for additional research regarding the use of physical restraint and seclusion with students across all settings.

White Papers* from which these recommendations are drawn:

Council for Children with Behavior Disorders (May, 2009). *CCBD Position on the Use of Physical Restraint Procedures in School Settings.* Reston, VA: Author.

Council for Children with Behavior Disorders (May, 2009). *CCBD Position on the Use of Seclusion Procedures in School Settings.* Reston, VA: Author.

End Notes

[1] Ryan, J. B., Peterson, R. L. Tetreault, G. & van der Hagen, E. (2007). Reducing the use of seclusion and restraint in a day school program. In M. A. Nunno, L. Bullard, & D. M. Day eds. *For our own good: Examining the Safety of High-Risk Interventions for Children and Young People.* (pp. 201-21 6) Washington, DC: Child Welfare League of America.

[2] Ryan, J.B., Robbins, K., Peterson, R.L. & Rozalski, M. (in press). Review of State Policies Concerning the Use of Physical Restraint Procedures in Schools. *Education and Treatment of Children.*

[3] Ryan, J. B., Peterson, R. L., & Rozalski, M. E. (2007). State policies concerning the use of seclusion timeout in schools. *Education and Treatment of Children, 30*(3), 215-239.

*Available from: Susan Fread Albrecht, Ed.D., NCSP; Assistant Professor, Department of Special Education; CCBD Advocacy and Governmental Relations Chair; Teachers College, Ball State University, Muncie, IN 47306; 765-285-5707; 765-285-4280 (fax); sfalbrecht@bsu.edu

In: Time Out: Examining Seclusion and... ISBN: 978-1-60876-932-2
Editor: Laura E. Kentley

Chapter 6

TESTIMONY OF TONI PRICE, MOTHER OF CEDRIC NAPOLEON

Toni Price

Thank you, Chairman Miller and the Committee, for holding this hearing today and inviting me to share my story with you.

My name is Toni Price. I am a foster mother, and Cedric was my foster son.

By the time Cedric came to my home at the age of 12, he'd been through a lot in his short life. His parents neglected him and his siblings and abused them both physically and emotionally. They were underfed and food was withheld from them. Cedric, the oldest, used to go rummaging for food for himself and his siblings. He'd scavenge through trash cans. Cedric began stealing food, and was caught stealing from a grocery store. Never knowing when he'd have his next meal, food was something Cedric became very sensitive about.

At 9 years old, his parents lost parental rights to Cedric and his siblings. His aunt and grandmother had also lost their rights to guardianship. Cedric went to many foster homes but struggled. After a number of unsuccessful placements, Cedric was sent to a "boot camp" facility north of Killeen. Unfortunately, at this boot camp, he experienced more abuse. He had a prominent scar on his face from being beaten with a shovel by a boot camp supervisor. It was after that facility that he came to live with my family and me at the age of 12.

Despite his experiences, Cedric came to me with a smile. He was very jovial, and truly loved to smile. He liked to bike, go bowling, and feed the ducks in a pond near our house. When he had extra energy, he loved to run to the end of our driveway and back. He got along well with the other children in the house, particularly my son, because he'd always wanted a big brother. They played a lot of basketball together. I remember at church Cedric wanted to be in a play, but there were no parts for him. He got this big smile on his face and said: "I know a part!" and went and stood on the stage. The director said "okay, you can be an angel." I knew he was sensitive about food, so I said he could have anything in the kitchen, he just had to tell me.

Cedric had behavioral problems, but they were never physical and he was never aggressive. We were able to find solutions to his misbehaving that worked. Once he stole a bag of chips from the kitchen. I made him pay me back. It was a consequence that worked. He didn't like parting with his allowance, and learned his lesson about stealing. But it was a consequence that didn't bring any of his previous abuse up to the surface. His therapist asked him once to describe a safe place. His answer was in a cave with solid rock walls, a steel door, and lots of food. Even though he was well fed at my home, food was a trigger for Cedric from the trauma of his childhood.

Cedric enrolled in a public middle school. He was placed in a class for students with behavioral problems. His first year in the school, in seventh grade, he had no problems. I didn't get phone calls, and he did well in school.

His eighth grade year, with a different teacher, he had a number of problems. He did not get along with the teacher, and would always say to me "I don't think this teacher likes me." I'd reassure him that she did. I got frequent calls from his teacher that year about verbal aggression, though I never got calls about physical aggression. I would ask the teacher to put Cedric on the phone and say: "Cedric, you know you have to do your work." He'd say: "yes ma'am." Sometimes Cedric would get in trouble at school for stealing food. But what I learned later was that in his classroom he was being withheld food as punishment for acting out.

The morning of his death, Cedric was put on what the teacher called a "delayed lunch" because he stopped working around 11am. This was, apparently, a common punishment for him. At 1pm Cedric got in more trouble when, still not having lunch, he was caught trying to steal candy. After 2:30, he still hadn't been allowed to eat his lunch, and got up to leave the classroom. After Cedric attempted to leave the classroom, he refused to sit back down in his chair so his teacher forced him into his chair and restrained him. She is roughly six feet tall and weighs over two hundred thirty pounds. Cedric was short- he was a little boy.

Cedric struggled as he was being held in his chair, so the teacher put him in a face down, or in a prone restraint, and sat on him. He struggled and said repeatedly: "I can't breathe." "If you can speak, you can breathe," she snapped at him. Shortly after that, he stopped speaking and he stopped struggling. He stopped moving at all. The teacher continued to restrain him. Finally the teacher and aide put Cedric back in his chair. The aide wiped drool off his mouth and they sat him up. But he slumped over and slipped out of his chair. Precious minutes passed by before a nurse was called.

I received a call at work that Cedric was not breathing and that an ambulance had been called. I rushed up to the school, not completely clear what was going on or what had happened. When I got to the school, my son was lying on the floor with a paramedic beside him. I knelt down and said: "Cedric, get up. You're not going to be in any trouble." But Cedric didn't move, and instead, the paramedic stood me up. My son was dead.

I didn't know the school was practicing restraint techniques on Cedric. I didn't know they were withholding food as a form of punishment. In fact, when I initially enrolled him at the school, I told administrators he'd been withheld food as a child and it was traumatic. When this teacher was having trouble with Cedric, I told her about my techniques with handling him at home. I tried to help her because Cedric was not a bad kid. He had come so far, and had such success in the seventh grade. I knew that he could be successful in the eighth.

The school never held meetings with me to address any behavioral problems. Aside from calls from his teacher, I didn't know the extent to which Cedric was getting in trouble and what they were doing to him. After his death, nobody from the school came for calling hours. The superintendent and the principal of the school wrote a letter of condolence. Nobody offered any help because I was just a foster mother. Days later, the teacher called, and my husband answered the phone. But instead of a heartfelt apology, she explained that she was just doing her job. She showed no sympathy, no compassion, no guilt.

This teacher took a child's life. But she also caused a lot of damage to his classmates, many of who were victims of trauma already. Those kids who witnessed it already had behavioral problems. His classmates and their parents were forbidden to talk to me. But for many of the children, witnessing the abuse of Cedric was so traumatic for them that they spoke, and in turn, their parents spoke to me.

After I read the autopsy report, I was taken aback at how much a school can get away with. Cedric's death was ruled a homicide. The school policy allows for "therapeutic floor holds" when a child is endangering himself or others. Here Cedric was not endangering himself or others. This floor hold should not have been done.

The teacher's previous treatment was reviewed and no problems were found with her conduct. No legal action was taken against this teacher, and as a foster mother, I didn't have the right to press charges.

Eventually a judge found this teacher's actions to be reckless, and Cedric's death not an accident. But she never received a criminal record or any kind of sentence. She was placed on a Texas registry for being abusive to children. But that registry only applies to Texas, and I have been told that this teacher now teaches at a public high school in Northern Virginia. Her Virginia teaching license shows her credentials to be K-12 special education. If that teacher was just doing her job, then something is very wrong with the system.

If I'd treated Cedric that way at home, I'd be in jail.

I want to make sure this doesn't happen to anyone else's child. It is awful the way Cedric died. He was a good kid. This should have never happened. The morning Cedric died, as he was boarding the bus, he turned around and got a beaming smile on his face, and said to me "you know I love you, ma."

He was a good kid.

In: Time Out: Examining Seclusion and... ISBN: 978-1-60876-932-2
Editor: Laura E. Kentley

Chapter 7

SECLUSIONS AND RESTRAINTS: SELECTED CASES OF DEATH AND ABUSE AT PUBLIC AND PRIVATE SCHOOLS AND TREATMENT CENTERS*

D. Gregory Kutz

WHY GAO DID THIS STUDY

GAO recently testified before the Committee regarding allegations of death and abuse at residential programs for troubled teens. Recent reports indicate that vulnerable children are being abused in other settings. For example, one report on the use of restraints and seclusions in schools documented cases where students were pinned to the floor for hours at a time, handcuffed, locked in closets, and subjected to other acts of violence. In some of these cases, this type of abuse resulted in death.

Given these reports, the Committee asked GAO to (1) provide an overview of seclusions and restraint laws applicable to children in public and private schools, (2) verify whether allegations of student death and abuse from the use of these methods are widespread, and (3) examine the facts and

---

* This is an edited, reformatted and augmented version of a U. S. Government Accountability Office publication dated May 2009.

circumstances surrounding cases where a student died or suffered abuse as a result of being secluded or restrained.

GAO reviewed federal and state laws and abuse allegations from advocacy groups, parents, and the media from the past two decades. GAO did not evaluate whether using restraints and seclusions can be beneficial. GAO examined documents related to closed cases, including police and autopsy reports and school policies. GAO also interviewed parents, attorneys, and school officials and conducted searches to determine the current employment status of staff involved in the cases.

View GAO-09-719T or key components. For more information, contact Gregory Kutz at (202) 512-6722 or kutzg@gao.gov.

What GAO Found

GAO found no federal laws restricting the use of seclusion and restraints in public and private schools and widely divergent laws at the state level. Although GAO could not determine whether allegations were widespread, GAO did find hundreds of cases of alleged abuse and death related to the use of these methods on school children during the past two decades. Examples of these cases include a 7 year old purportedly dying after being held face down for hours by school staff, 5 year olds allegedly being tied to chairs with bungee cords and duct tape by their teacher and suffering broken arms and bloody noses, and a 13 year old reportedly hanging himself in a seclusion room after prolonged confinement. Although GAO continues to receive new allegations from parents and advocacy groups, GAO could not find a single Web site, federal agency, or other entity that collects information on the use of these methods or the extent of their alleged abuse.

GAO also examined the details of 10 restraint and seclusion cases in which there was a criminal conviction, a finding of civil or administrative liability, or a large financial settlement. The cases share the following common themes: they involved children with disabilities who were restrained and secluded, often in cases where they were not physically aggressive and their parents did not give consent; restraints that block air to the lungs can be deadly; teachers and staff in the cases were often not trained on the use of seclusions and restraints; and teachers and staff from at least 5 of the 10 cases continue to be employed as educators. The table contains information on four of these cases.

Examples of Case Studies GAO Examined

Victim information	School	Case details
Male, 14, diagnosed with post traumatic stress	Texas public school	• 230 lb. teacher placed 129 lb. child facedown on floor and lay on top of him because he did not stay seated in class, causing his death. • Death ruled a homicide but grand jury did not indict teacher. Teacher currently teaches in Virginia.
Female, 4, born with cerebral palsy and diagnosed as autistic	West Virginia public school	• Child suffered bruising and post traumatic stress disorder after teachers restrained her in a wooden chair with leather straps— described as resembling a miniature electric chair—for being "uncooperative." • School board found liable for negligent training and supervision; teachers were found not liable, and one still works at the school.
Five victims, gender not disclosed, aged 6 and 7	Florida public school	• Volunteer teacher's aide, on probation for burglary and cocaine possession, gagged and duct-taped children for misbehaving. • No records that school did background check or trained aide. • Aide pled guilty to false imprisonment and battery.
Male, 9, diagnosed with a learning disability	New York public school	• Parents allowed school to use time out room only as a "last resort," but school put child in room repeatedly for hours at a time for offenses such as whistling, slouching, and hand waving. • Mother reported that the room smelled of urine and child's hands became blistered while trying to escape. • Jury awarded family $1,000 for each time child was put in the room.

Sources: Records including police reports, court documents, and interviews.

Mr. Chairman and Members of the Committee:

Thank you for the opportunity to discuss the use of restraints and seclusions on children and teens in public and private schools and selected treatment centers. In the context of this testimony, a restraint is defined as any manual method, physical or mechanical device, material, or equipment that immobilizes or reduces the ability of an individual to move his or her arms, legs, body, or head freely. Seclusion is the involuntary confinement of an individual alone in a room or area from which the individual is physically prevented from leaving.[1]

In certain circumstances, teachers and other staff may decide that it is necessary to restrain or seclude children in order to protect them from harming themselves or others. For example, some doctors and teachers contend that using seclusions and restraints can reduce injury and agitation and that it would be very difficult for organizations to run programs for children and adults with special needs without being able to use these methods. However, GAO has previously testified that these techniques can be dangerous because they may involve physical struggling, pressure on the chest, or other interruptions in breathing.[2] We found that children are subjected to restraint or seclusion at higher rates than adults and are at greater risk of injury. Even if no physical injury is sustained, we also testified that individuals can be severely traumatized during restraint. In addition, as part of our prior investigations of residential programs for troubled youth, we highlighted cases where staff at some programs employed unsafe restraint techniques, resulting in the death and abuse of teens in their care.[3] Recent reports by advocacy groups indicate that similar restraint techniques have been used at public and private school throughout the country. For example, in January 2009, the National Disability Rights Network issued a report documenting dozens of instances where students with disabilities were abusively pinned to the floor for hours at a time, handcuffed, locked in closets, and subjected to other traumatizing acts of violence. Just a few weeks ago, the Council of Parent Attorneys and Advocates, an organization that works to protect the civil rights of children with disabilities, issued a report describing similar examples of injury and abuse. In some of the cases described in these reports, the restraints and seclusions resulted in death.

Given these prior reports and testimony, you asked us to (1) provide an overview of federal and state laws related to the use of restraints and seclusions in public and private schools; (2) verify whether allegations of student death and abuse from the use of these techniques are widespread; and (3) examine the facts and circumstances surrounding selected criminal, civil, or administrative cases where a student died or suffered abuse as a result of being secluded or restrained.

To conduct our work, we first searched for all federal and state laws pertaining to the use of seclusions and restraints in public and private schools. To verify whether allegations of student death, injury, and abuse from the use of these techniques are widespread, we gathered available data on allegations made over the last two decades by interviewing relevant experts and officials from state agencies; performing extensive Internet and LexisNexis searches; reviewing federal and state court documents related to civil and criminal litigation; and seeking leads from state investigators, agency officials, attorneys, and parent advocacy groups. Except for the case studies discussed below, we did not attempt to verify the facts related to the allegations we reviewed, nor did we attempt to evaluate cases where the use of restraints and seclusions may have been necessary or beneficial.

To select our case studies, we searched for restraint and seclusion cases from the last two decades in which there was a criminal conviction, finding of civil or administrative liability, or a large financial settlement. As part of the selection process, we focused on cases involving children from public and private schools or treatment programs in which residents attended classes; we excluded cases involving children in psychiatric facilities or juvenile detention centers. Ultimately, we selected 10 cases from 9 different states for further review. To the extent possible, we conducted interviews with related parties, including current and former school staff and officials, attorneys and law enforcement officials, and the parents of the victims. We also attempted to obtain training policies on restraints and seclusions followed at each school and treatment center involved in the cases. Further, where applicable, we reviewed police reports; witness statements; autopsy reports; state agency oversight reviews and investigations; and court documents, including trial transcripts, depositions, and plaintiffs' complaints and defendants' answers. We also conducted searches to determine whether the individuals who restrained or secluded the children in our case studies had previous criminal histories and whether they are still teaching or working with children. Finally, in addition to the 10 new cases we selected for this testimony, we also included 3 cases involving the use of face down restraints from our previous work on residential treatment programs for troubled youth. We performed our work from February 2009 to April 2009 in accordance with standards prescribed by the Council of Inspectors General for Integrity and Efficiency (CIGIE).

Overview of Federal and State Laws Related to the Use of Restraints and Seclusions

Overall, we found no federal regulations related to seclusions and restraints in public and private schools and widely divergent laws at the state level. We also identified at least five states that currently collect and report information related to the use of seclusions and restraints in public and private schools.

At the federal level, the Children's Health Act of 2000 amended Title V of the Public Health Service Act to regulate the use of restraints and seclusions on residents of certain hospitals and health care facilities that receive any type of federal funds as well as on children in certain residential, non-medical, community-based facilities that receive funds under the Public Health Service Act. CMS has issued additional regulations regarding the use of restraints and seclusions on patients of hospitals that participate in the Medicare and Medicaid programs. However, there are no federal laws restricting the use of restraints and seclusion in public or private schools. With regard to children with disabilities, the Individuals with Disabilities Education Act (IDEA) requires that eligible students be educated in the least restrictive environment. IDEA also mandates that special education students have an Individualized Education Program (IEP), a written document that in part explains the educational goals of the student and the types of services to be provided. IEPs are developed by parents and school personnel and may contain instructions related to the use of strategies to support the student. These could include, for example, instruction approaches and behavioral interventions such as the use of seclusion and restraints.

Furthermore, state laws and regulations in this area vary widely. For example, nineteen states have no laws or regulations related to the use of seclusions or restraints in schools.[4] Other states have regulations, but they may only apply to selected schools in certain situations. For example, seven states place some restrictions of the use of restraints, but do not regulate seclusions.[5] Seventeen states require that selected staff receive training before being permitted to restrain children.[6] Thirteen states require schools to obtain consent prior to using foreseeable or non- emergency physical restraints,[7] while nineteen require parents to be notified after restraints have been used.[8] Two states require annual reporting on the use of restraints.[9] Eight states specifically prohibit the use of prone restraints or restraints that impede a child's ability to breathe.[10] For an overview of applicable seclusion and restraint laws and regulations in all fifty states and the District of Columbia, see appendix 1. In addition to these legal requirements, we found at least four states that are currently collecting and reporting information from school districts on the use of restraints and seclusions, including Kansas, Pennsylvania, Texas, and Rhode Island.

ALLEGATIONS OF DEATH AND ABUSE RELATED TO THE USE OF SECLUSIONS AND RESTRAINTS AT PUBLIC AND PRIVATE SCHOOLS

Although we could not determine whether allegations of death and abuse were widespread, we did discover hundreds of such allegations at public and private schools across the nation between the years 1990 and 2009.[11] Almost all of the allegations we identified involved children with disabilities.[12] While this number represents a small share of all children in public and private schools nationwide over these years, these allegations raise serious issues for a significant number of children, families, and those entrusted with their education and care. Although we continue to receive new allegations from parents and advocacy groups, we could not locate a single Web site, federal agency, or other entity that collects comprehensive information on this issue. For example, the Department of Education's Office of Civil Rights receives complaints about the inappropriate use of restraint and seclusion on children with disabilities, but officials said their case management system does not have the ability to single such complaints out for tabulation. In addition, the Department of Health and Human Services funds the collection of information about investigations conducted by state child protective services agencies through the National Child Abuse and Neglect Data System, but it does not have a code to indicate whether perpetrators are teachers or staff at public and private schools.

It is important to emphasize that allegations should not be confused with proof of actual abuse. However, in terms of meeting our objective, the hundreds of allegations we found came from a number of sources, including our own research, advocacy groups, news accounts, parents, and attorneys. We often identified multiple allegations from each of our sources; for example, an attorney based in South Carolina said his office has worked on at least 15 school cases involving the restraint and seclusion of children during the last 3 years, including a student's being shut in a classroom closet. Other examples of death and abuse claims are as follows; we do not know the outcomes of these cases.

- A 13-year-old boy with attention deficit hyperactivity disorder at an alternative public school hung himself in a seclusion room weeks after threatening to commit suicide, using a cord a teacher reportedly provided him to hold up his pants.

- A 7-year-old girl died at a private day treatment center after being held for hours in a face-down, or prone, restraint on the floor by multiple staff members. The staff was allegedly unaware she had stopped breathing until they rolled her limp body over and discovered she had begun to turn blue.
- A 9-year-old boy in foster care died at a public charter school after his teacher took him to a "time out" room and restrained him using a "basket hold," which in this case was described as an adult standing behind a child, holding the child's crossed arms and taking him to the floor. Purportedly, the boy began to make a noise like he was vomiting, then slumped over after being released. The teacher testified that she initially thought he was playing dead and joked with other staffers about planning his funeral.
- A 17-year-old boy reportedly died from an asthma attack while being restrained by a counselor at a private school for emotionally disturbed teens.
- Disabled children as young as 6 years old were allegedly placed in strangleholds, restrained for extended periods of time, confined to dark rooms, prevented from using the restroom causing them to urinate on themselves, and tethered to ropes in one public school district.
- A special education teacher at a public school was accused of using bungee cords and duct tape to fasten children as young as 5 years old to chairs designed to support kids with muscular difficulties. According to parents, their children sustained injuries such as broken arms and bloody noses while in this teacher's class. A teacher's aide told investigators that the woman used the restraints on a daily basis to punish the children.
- According to the father of an 8-year-old autistic boy, his son suffered from scratches, bruises and a broken nose after being put in a prone restraint by his public school teacher and aide.
- A sixth-grade special education student reportedly had his leg broken by the public school teacher who was trying to restrain him.
- A 12-year-old girl allegedly had her arm fractured by a special education teacher who put her in a "therapeutic hold," described as being similar to a "bear hug" or hold a student's arms behind their back.

- An autistic student at a public school claims he was strapped with his pants pulled down onto a toilet training chair for hours at a time over several days.

In addition, we were able to obtain data showing that thousands of public and private school students were restrained or secluded during the last academic year. These data do not show the inappropriate use of restraints and seclusions, but rather the number of times the techniques were used during an academic year. Specifically, Texas and California, two states that together contain more than 20 percent of the nation's children, collect self-reported information from school officials on the use of these methods. Texas public school officials stated they restrained 4,202 students 18,741 times during the September 2007 through June 2008 academic year. During the same time period, California officials reported 14,354 instances of students' being subjected to restraint, seclusion or other undefined "emergency interventions" in public and private schools. Other states that currently collect and report this type of information include Kansas, Pennsylvania, and Rhode Island, but we did not obtain data from these states.

Cases of Death and Abuse Related to the Use of Restraints and Seclusions

Children, especially those with disabilities, are reportedly being restrained and secluded in public and private schools and other facilities, sometimes resulting in injury and death. The 10 closed cases we examined illustrate the following themes: (1) children with disabilities were sometimes restrained and secluded even when they did not appear to be physically aggressive and their parents did not give consent; (2) facedown or other restraints that block air to the lungs can be deadly; (3) teachers and staff in these cases were often not trained in the use of restraints and techniques; and (4) teachers and staff from these cases continue to be employed as educators. In addition to the 10 cases we identified for this testimony, 3 cases from our previous testimonies on residential treatment programs for troubled youth also show that face down restraints, or those that impede respiration, can be deadly.

Case Studies from Current Investigation

For our current investigation, we identified 10 seclusion and restraint cases occurring at public and private schools and selected treatment centers over the past two decades. Common themes related to the cases studies are as follows:

Children with Disabilities: Although we did not specifically limit the scope of our investigation to incidents involving disabled children, most the hundreds of allegations we identified related to children with disabilities. In addition, 9 of our 10 closed cases involve children with disabilities or a history of troubled behavior. The children in these cases were diagnosed with autism or other conditions, including post traumatic stress disorder and attention deficit hyperactivity disorder. Although we did not evaluate whether the seclusion and restraint used by the staff in our cases was proper under applicable state laws, we did observe that the children in the cases were restrained or secluded as disciplinary measures, even when their behavior did not appear to be physically aggressive. For example, teachers restrained a 4 year old with cerebral palsy in a device that resembled a miniature electric chair because she was reportedly being "uncooperative." In other cases, we found that teachers and other staff did not have parental consent prior to using restraints and seclusions. For example, an IEP for a 9 year old with learning disabilities specified that placement in a timeout room could be used to correct inappropriate behavior, but only as a last resort. However, teachers confined this child to a small, dirty room 75 times over the course of 6 months for offenses such as whistling, slouching, and hand waving. Parents in another case gave a teacher explicit instructions to stop restraining their 7-year-old child and secluding her for prolonged periods of time. Despite these instructions, the restraints and seclusions continued. In another case, a residential day school implemented a behavior plan, without parental consent, that included confining an 11-year-old autistic child to his room for extended periods of time, restricting his food, and using physical restraints. The child was diagnosed with post traumatic stress disorder as a result of this treatment. Currently, thirteen states require schools to obtain consent prior to using foreseeable or non-emergency physical restraints.[13]

Death from Face Down Restraints or Restraints that Block the Airway: Of the hundreds of allegations we identified, at least 20 involved restraints that resulted in death. Of the 10 closed cases we examined, 4 involved children who died as a result of being restrained. In all 4 cases, staff members used restraint techniques that restricted the flow of air to the child's lungs. In one of these cases, an aide sat on top of a child to prevent him from being disruptive and ultimately smothered him. The other cases related to the use of different types of prone restraints, a technique that typically involves one or more staff members holding a child face down on the floor. Although some of the teachers and staff involved in these cases were trained on the use of prone restraints, the children in their care still died as a result of its use. However, we did not attempt to evaluate the types of training they received or whether they actually implemented the procedure according to the training. Currently, eight states specifically prohibit the use of prone restraints or restraints that impede a child's ability to breathe.[14]

Untrained Staff: Although we did not evaluate specific training methods, evidence we gathered suggests that the teachers and other staff involved in our 10 closed cases were often not trained in the use of restraints. For example, staff involved in the death of a child in one case acknowledged that they were inadequately trained. A principal in another case testified that she did not know whether a substitute teacher who taped children to their chairs to make them sit still had ever been provided with the school policy on restraint. A local school board in a fourth case was found civilly liable for negligently supervising and training teachers after a 4-year-old girl was strapped to a chair for allegedly being uncooperative. A school district agreed to implement policy changes to improve training in a fifth case as part of a settlement agreement after a teacher repeatedly restrained a frail 7 year old. Lastly, in a sixth case, a volunteer teacher's aid with a history of armed burglary and cocaine possession was allowed to tape first graders to a blackboard and seal their mouths shut; we found no evidence that the school trained this aide or even conducted a background check on her before letting her into the classroom. Currently, seventeen states require that staff receive training before being permitted to restrain children.[15]

Continued Employment in Education: Although we did not evaluate specific state licensing requirements, we did observe that in at least 5 of our cases, the teachers or other staff involved in the injurious restraint or seclusion of children continued to work with students or had licenses to do so. For example, a 230 pound teacher in Texas who fatally restrained a 129 pound teenage boy facedown on a mat currently works as a public high school teacher in Virginia. The Texas Department of Family Protective Services

(DFPS) placed the teacher's name on a Texas registry that lists individuals found to have abused or neglected children. An administrative law judge later ruled that the woman used unnecessary force on the special education student, sustained the DFPS's abuse finding, and affirmed that the teacher's information should be released through the registry. Despite this listing, she is currently licensed in Virginia to instruct children with disabilities. In another example, the assistant principal who fatally restrained a child after holding him facedown on the floor for approximately an hour currently works as a principal at another public school in the same district. In addition, one of the teachers who strapped the 4-year-old child to a chair for allegedly being uncooperative still teaches at the school where the incident occurred, while the teacher who repeatedly restrained the frail 7 year old left her school but immediately began teaching in another district in the same state. Finally, the substitute teacher who taped children to their chairs and was found guilty of unlawful restraint and battery in July 2008 still holds a state substitute teaching certificate, which does not expire until June 2009.

Table 1 provides a summary of the cases we examined; a more detailed narrative on each of the cases follows the table.

Table 1. Summary of Case Studies

Case	Student information	Location and type of institution	Year of incident (s)	Case details
1	Male, 14, had a history of disruptive behavior	Pennsylvania; private, nonprofit residential treatment center	1998	• Two staff members trained in the use of restraints pinned the student facedown on the floor for 20 minutes after he tried to attack a counselor. • Student died from a brain injury as a result of a lack of oxygen. • Death ruled an accident and no criminal charges were filed. • Facility settled with student's mother for over $1 million with no admission of liability. Pennsylvania banned prone restraints in 2008.

Table 1. (Continued)

Case	Student information	Location and type of institution	Year of incident (s)	Case details
2	Male, 14, diagnosed with post traumatic stress and other disorders	2002 Texas; public school		• 230 lb. special education teacher placed 129 lb. student into a prone restraint and lay on top of him because he would not stay seated. • Student died as a result of compression of the trunk. • Death ruled a homicide, but no criminal charges filed. • Teacher currently teaches in Virginia and is licensed to instruct children with disabilities.
3	Male, from the age of 11 through 13, diagnosed as mentally retarded and autistic	New York; private residential school and state facility for children with developmental disabilities	2004 and 2007	• Case involves two residential facilities • Without notifying parents, child "ignored" and secluded in his room for extended periods of time at first facility and had access to regular meals restricted. • Parents removed child from the school alleging neglect; case resulted in state law granting parents full access to investigative records in abuse cases. • At second facility, student died by suffocation after an aide sat on top of him because he was being disruptive while riding in a van. • The aide and driver of the van stopped at a game store and one of the employee's houses while the child lay unconscious in the backseat. • The aide was convicted of manslaughter and is currently in prison.

Table 1. (Continued)

Case	Student information	Location and type of institution	Year of incident (s)	Case details
4	Male, 15, diagnosed as autistic	Michigan , public school	2003	• Student suffered a seizure and lost control of his extremities and bladder and later became uncooperative. • Assistant principal and other staff did not provide medical attention for the seizure and instead placed student in a prone restraint for approximately an hour, resulting in death. • Death ruled an accident and no criminal charges filed. • Mother settled a civil suit with the school district for $1.3 million. • Assistant principal is now a principal at another school in the district.
5	Female, 4, born with cerebral palsy and diagnosed as autistic	West Virginia; public school	1998	• Child was "uncooperative," so teachers restrained her in a chair with multiple leather straps that resembled a "miniature electric chair." • Child suffered bruising, wet the bed, and had temper tantrums. Doctor later diagnosed child with post traumatic stress syndrome. • Jury in civil case did not find teachers liable for any wrongdoing but found school board liable for negligent supervision and training in the use of restraints and awarded the family $460,000. • West Virginia has since banned the use of restraints on pre-kindergarten children. • At least one of the three teachers responsible for the

Table 1. (Continued)

Case	Student information	Location and type of institution	Year of incident (s)	Case details
				restraint still teaches at the school.
6	Four males under 6, all in special education class and one diagnosed with a condition similar to Down syndrome.	Tennessee public school	2003 to 2004	• To prevent a child with a Down syndrome-type condition from wandering, the teacher used sheets to strap the boy to a cot while he was wearing a 5lb., lead physical therapy vest. • The teacher also hit the children with a flyswatter, a ruler, and her hand. • Teacher pleaded guilty to felony child abuse, neglect, and misdemeanor assault and was placed on 3 years probation.
7	Male, 8, diagnosed with attention deficit hyperactivity disorder	Illinois public school	2006	• Substitute restrained child to a chair with masking tape and also taped his mouth shut because the boy would not remain seated. • Substitute found guilty of unlawful restraint and aggravated battery. He was sentenced to 2 years probation, community service, and a psychological evaluation. • Substitute still possesses an Illinois substitute teaching certificate, which expires in June 2009.
8	Five students, gender not disclosed, aged 6 and 7	Florida public school	2003	• Volunteer teacher's aide, a felon on probation for armed burglary, grand theft and cocaine possession, gagged and duct-taped children to their desks as punishment for misbehaving. • There is no record that the school trained aide or conducted a background

Table 1. (Continued)

Case	Student information	Location and type of institution	Year of incident (s)	Case details
				check before allowing aide into the class room. • Aide pled guilty to false imprisonment and battery, was placed on 5 years probation, and ordered to attend anger management classes. • Aide was later arrested again for possession of cocaine.
9	Female, 7, diagnosed with Asperger's syndrome, a form of autism	California public school	2001 to 2002	• Teacher secluded child in a walled off area because she refused to do work, sat on top of her because she was wiggling a loose tooth, and repeatedly restrained and abused her. • The student was awarded $260,000 in a civil settlement, although the school and teacher did not admit liability. • Teacher left the school but began teaching again in a different school district.
10	Male, 9, diagnosed with a learning disability	New York public school	1992 to 1993	• School was only supposed to use timeout room as a last resort to correct inappropriate behavior but put child in the room 75 times over a 6 month period for hours at a time for offenses such as whistling, slouching, and hand waving. • The room was unlocked, but a staff person would hold it shut to prevent the child from leaving; the child's hands became blistered while trying to escape.

Table 1. (Continued)

Case	Student information	Location and type of institution	Year of incident (s)	Case details
				• Mother reported that the room was dirty and smelled of urine. • A jury in a civil suit awarded family $75,000: $1,000 for every time the child was placed in the room.

Source: Records including police reports, court documents, and interviews.

Case 1: The student was a 14 year old male. He was living in a private, non-profit, residential treatment center for troubled children in Pennsylvania and attending a private school operated by the center when he died in 1998 as a result of being physically restrained. He had been placed in the custody of the non-profit by the New Jersey Department of Youth and Family Services in 1995.

According to a report by the District Attorney, on December 10, 1998, following a fight with a fellow student at a school on the treatment center's campus, the 14 year old returned to his dormitory room. A 195 pound male counselor entered the room to counsel the 125 pound boy about the fight. The boy was agitated and attempted to stab the counselor at least three times with a pen. To prevent further attack, the counselor applied a prone restraint in which the boy ended up face down on the floor with the counselor's left knee on the left side of his body and the counselor's right leg across his back. At this point, the boy no longer had the pen in his hand. The counselor locked the boy's arms behind his back. A female counselor heard the boy say, "I'm sorry I hit you" and "I hate you all." While being physically restrained on the floor, the boy continued to yell, kick, and struggle. A 155 pound male counselor also entered the room and placed a vinyl mat under the boy's head to prevent injury. The treatment center's records reveal that the boy had previously been physically restrained 17 times. The treatment center would not release the boy's treatment plan.

After approximately 12 minutes, the 195 pound counselor became tired and the 155 pound counselor took his place, locking the boy's arms behind the boy's back and positioning his body so that it lay off to the left side of the boy. The 155 pound counselor physically restrained the boy for approximately 8 minutes during which time the boy continued to struggle and scream "Get the [expletive] off me, get off me." Another child reported hearing the boy yell, "Stop it, I can't breathe." The 195 pound counselor responded, "You'll be able to breathe if you stop struggling." After approximately 20 minutes of physical restraint, the student lost consciousness, and CPR was administered. The boy was taken to the hospital where he died a day later. The autopsy determined the cause of death as hypoxic encephalopathy due to compressional asphyxia, a brain injury sustained as a result of lack of oxygen due to the compression of the student's chest.

Each of the counselors who applied the restraint that led to the boy's death were trained and certified in applying physical restraints. According to an instruction manual, employees at the center were trained in applying multiple restraints, two of which required the student to remain face down on the floor in a prone position. In his report, the District Attorney concluded that the treatment center's policy did not appear to have any inherent flaw in the technique and that the policy was well designed and appeared to have been followed by all the counselors involved. The coroner ruled that the death was accidental and the District Attorney did not file charges against the counselors.

In May 1999, the boy's mother sued the treatment center and two of the counselors who applied the restraint that led to the boy's death, alleging negligence. She claimed that the counselors used excessive force, and that the treatment center did not adequately train their counselors to deal with respiratory distress during a physical restraint. The defendants denied these allegations and said the restraint was employed for the protection of everyone involved in the situation. The counselors further stated that they acted with due care and safety of the boy.

In May 2006, before the case went to trial, the boy's mother, the treatment center, and the two counselors reached a settlement. According to the terms of the settlement, the boy's mother would be paid over $1 million. The treatment center and the two counselors did not admit any liability in the boy's death as part of this settlement. The two counselors who physically restrained the boy did not have criminal histories. They no longer work at the treatment center, but we were unable to determine whether they currently counsel children.

In October 1999, less than a year after the boy's death, the Pennsylvania Department of Public Welfare enacted regulations that prohibit child residential facilities and day treatment centers from administering restraints that apply pressure or weight on a child's respiratory system. Consequently, we requested the treatment center provide its current policies and training manuals regarding restraints. In response, the treatment center sent us a letter stating it no longer uses prone restraints. In addition, it provided us a copy of its policy allowing physical restraints in residential treatment facilities and education programs and a workbook used to obtain certification in physical restraints. The center's policy states trained staff members are authorized to use physical restraint methods. According to the workbook, staff can apply physical force that reduces or restricts mobility while an individual is in an upright or seated position, lying face up, or in the transport of an individual from one location to another.

Case 2: The victim was a 14-year-old male who died in 2002 from being restrained by his middle school teacher at a public school in Texas. He was taken from his family at the age of nine after the Texas Department of Family and Protective Services (TDFPS)[16] received reports that the boy and his siblings were being neglected and emotionally and physically abused, according to his foster care records. He described having to feed himself by taking food from trash cans and grocery stores. He was placed in his last foster home after being hit in the head with a shovel at the residential treatment center where he resided. Less than a year before he died, he told his therapist that his idea of a safe place was a cave with solid rock walls, a steel door, and lots of food. His most recent psychological assessment noted that the boy suffered from posttraumatic stress disorder, conduct disorder, oppositional defiance disorder, attention deficit hyperactivity disorder, and narcissistic personality disorder. The child also had a fear of not being allowed to eat and often horded food as a result of his prior abuse, according to TDFPS. The boy was in a special education class that focused on behavior management. We were unable to obtain the child's individual education plan.

The day the child died, he had been denied his lunch by school staff as a form of punishment, according to an investigation by TDFPS. Reports differ on what prompted this disciplinary action. The classroom teacher told police she gave him a "delayed lunch" because he had stopped working at about 11 a.m. and started asking if he could eat. She said this was a common occurrence. A teacher's aide also told police that he placed the child on "delayed lunch" at about 1 p.m. after the boy tried to steal candy. The child became agitated at about 2:30 p.m. and left the classroom, according to TDFPS. The aide ran after the boy and brought him back to the classroom, but he would not remain seated. The teacher warned him to sit down at least twice before forcibly placing him in his chair. She told police that she used a "basket hold" restraint on him while he remained seated, standing behind him and grabbing his wrists so his arms crossed over his torso. He continued to struggle, so the teacher told police she rolled him onto a mat face down into a "therapeutic floor hold" and lay on top of him. A student said his arms were pinned beneath him. The child was 5 feet 1 inch tall and weighed 129 pounds. The teacher was about 6 feet tall and weighed in excess of 230 pounds. An aide, meanwhile, held the boy's feet. The boy kicked and cursed. He repeatedly said that he could not breathe and that he was going to pass out. Multiple witnesses told investigators that he also said, "I give." After the boy became silent, the teacher continued to restrain him. An assistant principal who had entered the classroom while the boy was still struggling asked the teacher to release him, saying 15 minutes had passed. School district policy required administrator approval for extending restraint past this time period. The teacher and an aide put the child's limp body back in his chair, and the aide wiped drool from his mouth. The assistant principal told police that they thought he had been "playing possum." Once the assistant principal noticed that the child was unresponsive, she said she asked for the school nurse. The nurse arrived and performed CPR while someone phoned 911. The child was taken to the hospital and pronounced dead. A dozen students in the classroom had witnessed the incident.

Medical examiners performed an autopsy and determined that the boy died from mechanical compression of the trunk. His death was ruled a homicide and local police investigated the incident for possible prosecution. During the investigation, the teacher told authorities that the school district trained her on how to restrain students. School policy stated that restraint can be used if the child is an immediate danger to himself or others or if the child is trying to exit the classroom with the intent to leave school premises. One school district restraint trainer told police that the teacher had a very difficult classroom—the worst in the district. She also said she had reviewed the teacher's previous "therapeutic floor holds" and found no problems with the way the teacher executed the procedure.

A grand jury decided not to take action on the boy's death. TDFPS launched their own investigation and found "reason to believe" the teacher physically abused the student on the day he died. TDFPS placed her name on the department's "Central Registry," which lists individuals found to have abused or neglected children. The teacher appealed the listing to the State Office of Administrative Hearings. An administrative law judge found that the child's actions prior to being restrained did not put himself or anyone else in danger. The judge also determined that the boy had already been returned to the classroom uneventfully. The judge also found that the teacher employed the restraint as an inappropriate disciplinary tactic, using excessive, unnecessary force out of proportion to the minimal risk posed by the child's action. The teacher also ignored pleas and warnings that the child could not breathe and continued to hold him after he became still and quiet, the judge noted. Under these circumstances, the judge determined the teacher's action to be reckless and the child's death not an accident. The judge sustained the department's abuse finding and allowed the information to continue to be released to upon request to officials responsible for children. The teacher does not have a criminal record and currently works as a teacher at a public high school in Virginia. Her Virginia teaching license lists endorsements for the instruction of students in grades K-12 who have specific learning disabilities, emotional disturbances and mental retardation. We have referred this matter to the Virginia Department of Education for further investigation.

Case 3: The student was 11 when he was first abused at a private facility in New York before being smothered to death 2 years later by an employee at a state facility who restrained him in a van. The child was non-verbal and had been diagnosed as mentally retarded and autistic.

In January 2003, the family enrolled the child at a private, nonprofit residential school paid for by Medicaid. According to his parents, they were struggling to toilet train their son and had heard the school had been very successful with these situations. Initially, he appeared to be doing well, successfully using the toilet about 50 percent of the time. In the summer and fall of 2004, the boy became increasingly more aggressive and began sporadically taking off his clothes. Without parental notification or consent, the school implemented an adjusted behavioral support plan,[17] called "planned ignore." As part of this plan, the child had restrictions placed on his access to regular meals. According to school documents, he was required to be dressed in order to eat his meals. If he did not get dressed after one prompt from the staff, he was not allowed to eat his meal and received only yogurt, milk, juice or water for breakfast, lunch, and dinner. State investigations subsequently found that in a 1 month timeframe, the child missed almost 40 percent of his regular meals. When the child refused to get dressed, he also was secluded in his room for extended periods of time, while an employee held the door closed. The child's isolation prevented him from participating in meals, school, and leisure activities. One staff member described the school's protocol for the student as "putting him in a dark hole and giving him nothing." During this time he missed approximately 2 weeks of classes. The school also suspended the family's visitation rights.

In October 2004, the father said he found his son disoriented and lying naked in his own urine. The window in his son's room was taped, pictures and toys had been removed and his son, noticeably thinner, was covered in bruises. Although the parents had not consented to any form of restraint being used against their son, school injury reports confirm that the staff did use physical restraint. The reports cite bruising and scrapes over the student's entire body, documenting the bruises as "too numerous to count." As a result, the parents removed their son from the school and took him home. The parents said their son seemed "emotionally damaged" and according to his psychiatrist, was suffering from post traumatic stress disorder.

As a result of allegations by the family, several New York state agencies and the district attorney's office initiated investigations of the abuse and of the school's regulatory compliance. Although the school was required to correct deficiencies of care identified in these investigations, no actions were taken against any of the staff involved in the incidents, and we were unable to determine whether the staff members are still working at the school. The parents then filed a complaint with the New York State Inspector General (IG) asking that it review the quality of the agencies' investigations. The IG ultimately found deficiencies related to each investigation and recommended, in part, that the relevant state agencies take steps to ensure that abuse cases are investigated thoroughly. The IG report further stated that there is no justification for a child in a private, state-certified facility to be afforded less protection from abuse than a child in a state run facility. In addition, the child's family worked to pass a state law, named in their son's honor, requiring parents or guardians to be notified within 24 hours of an incident that affects the health and safety of their child. The law, which became effective in 2007, also grants parents and guardians full access to records relevant to investigations of patient abuse and increases fines for state licensed facilities that do not comply with applicable rules and regulations.

Unfortunately, before this law was passed, the family suffered an even greater tragedy. In the fall of 2005, their son's emotional problems escalated. He was experiencing rages and, after several trips and weeks spent in the hospital, the family could still not stabilize his behavior. In October 2005, the child was transferred from an upstate New York hospital and placed in a state-operated facility for children with developmental disabilities.

Sixteen months later, the child was on a field trip when he began acting up and was smothered to death by one of the school's health aides. Police records indicate that during the van ride, the child got out of his seatbelt and began grabbing at another student. According to his parents, their son's behavior plan included the use of a seatbelt buckle guard, a device that prevents the wearer from disengaging the buckle. However, to their knowledge the buckle guard allegedly was not being used that day. Instead, one of the health aides got in the back seat of the van and first tried to restrain the child by pulling his arm's across his chest while he was in a seated wrap position. When that did not calm the child, the aide sat on the child. .. Although the family had consented to the use of some restraints against their son, this improper restraint caused the child to lose consciousness and stop breathing.

After the child fell unconscious, neither of the employees in the van performed CPR or first aid. Instead they continued to drive around, stopping at a game store and one of the employee's houses before finally going back to the school. In a statement made to police, the aide said "[he] realized that [the child] had stopped breathing when he stopped moving" but didn't call anyone for help because he and the other aide were afraid of losing their jobs and going to jail. The child had been unconscious for over 30 minutes when CPR rescue efforts first began. The autopsy report cites the cause of death as cardiorespiratory arrest due to compressive asphyxia. The aide responsible for smothering the child was convicted of second degree manslaughter and is scheduled to be released from prison in 2012.

Case 4: This 15-year-old male died on the first day of school in August 2003 after being restrained by staff at a Michigan public high school. The student had been previously diagnosed with autism and had an Individual Education Plan (IEP) signed by his mother that summer which stated that his disability affected his ability to perform socially or academically at his grade level. The plan described him as being inquisitive, artistic and motivated to please. It also stated that the boy enjoyed verbal praise and positive adult attention.

On the day of his death, an aide accompanied the student to a choir class with approximately 20 other students. In addition to the student, there was one other autistic student and three special education students. About 15 to 20 minutes into the class, the student's eyes rolled back into his head, his body began to convulse, and he lost control of his bladder. The aide stated that she believed the student was having a seizure. She placed the student on the floor and after several minutes, another aide pressed the room's emergency button. The school's assistant principal responded to the classroom and decided that the student did not need medical attention. He instructed another staff member to call the student's mother to pick him up.

Approximately 10 minutes after the seizure, the student got up but seemed unsteady so the instructional aide tried to assist him into a seated position. At this point, the student jumped up and began flailing his arms. The choir teacher, who had moved her students to another part of the room to continue the class, made another call for assistance and the assistant principal returned, this time accompanied by another aide. Shortly thereafter, the student began to scream and flail his arms again. According to the assistant principal's written statement, he believed that the student might hurt himself or others, so he and the two aides placed the student in a full restraint facedown on the floor. Specifically, the assistant principal was holding the student's arms behind his back, one of the aides held his legs down, and the other was holding his shoulders. The assistant principal went on to state that it was very difficult to hold onto the student and that every time they relaxed the restraint, he would begin to struggle again. They restrained him in this manner for approximately an hour, but did not call any medical professionals to attend to the student during this time.

The assistant principal and the aides eventually stopped the restraint when a man and woman who were friends of the mother arrived to pick the student up. The male friend tried to talk to the student but he did not respond. Both the assistant principal and the two friends thought the student looked strange and asked the school staff to call 911. The assistant principal checked the student and said he felt a pulse, but the female friend stated that he was not breathing. The assistant principal checked again for a pulse and found none, so the female friend started CPR. The assistant principal, who had an expired CPR certification, assisted by pinching the student's nose closed. Police and firefighters arrived and continued CPR for an additional 30 minutes until paramedics transported the student to a hospital, where he was pronounced dead. In the autopsy report, the medical examiner concluded that the student had suffered an apparent seizure and further wrote that "restraint in the prone position of emotionally and physically agitated individuals is recognized as being associated with sudden death, even without significant chest or neck compression." The official cause of death was listed as "prolonged physical restraint in prone position associated with extreme mental and motor agitation." His death was ruled an accident and no criminal charges were filed.

In 2006, the student's mother settled a civil case against the school district and the regional educational services agency for $1.3 million. In her deposition, the choir teacher stated that she had no idea the student was autistic until she saw him walk into the class with his aide and that she had no prior information on the student. In his deposition, the school's principal testified that neither he nor the assistant principal had received training about the dangers of restraining an individual on the floor. The aide who had held the student's feet to the floor also testified in a deposition that he was never given any advice or information on restraining students. Further, according to an instructor who had provided training that included the use of restraints to both the Regional Educational Service Agency (RESA) and school district staff testified, the instructional aide who accompanied the student into the class had last received such training in 1987. At the time of the incident, the instructor said that training, which includes the use of restraints, was offered to school district employees but the decision about who had to be trained was left to principals or program supervisors.

As of April 2009, the assistant principal who made the decision to restrain the student currently serves as the principal of the district's middle school and one of the other staff members who restrained the student is currently employed by the district's regional educational service agency. We were unable to determine whether the other staff members are still employed by this or any other school district. None of the staff members who restrained the child had any criminal histories.

As a result of this student's death, and another student death in 2003 caused by improper restraint, a member of the Michigan State Board of Education (SBE) told us that SBE changed its recommended policies on the use of restraints and seclusions. However, though the policy encourages local school districts to collect and report data on the use of these techniques to the Michigan Department of Education, the board member expressed doubt that this was actually done. In each year since the policy was enacted, the member said that she has requested any statistics or reports on the use of seclusion and restraints but has never received any information.

Case 5: The child in this case was an adopted, 4-year-old female who was strapped to a chair by her teacher at a West Virginia public school. The child was born with cerebral palsy and was later diagnosed with autism. In February 1998, she started special education classes and shortly thereafter, began to have tantrums and wet her pants at school. According to the child's mother, these behaviors continued at home and, even though the child was toilet trained. Her mother also said that the girl began coming home from school with bruises covering her calves, chest, and wrists.

According to the school and teachers, after the girl was enrolled in school for just 10 days, her mother arrived at school to pick her up and was told by a teacher's aide that she was being uncooperative and had been restrained in a chair for medically fragile children. The mother later claimed that, because the child was autistic, she would act up when she needed to use the bathroom. The school and teachers stated that they put her in the chair because she was "uncooperative." According to the mother, the chair resembled an electric chair and was high backed with multiple leather straps across the arms, chest, lap, and legs. The mother told the school to never use the chair again.

That same day, the child's mother removed her daughter from the West Virginia Elementary School and reported the bruises and use of the restraint to the State Board of Education. When the Board provided no help, the mother sued the school district alleging, among other things, that the school's actions directly and proximately caused and will continue to cause her daughter great psychological and emotional stress, developmental delays, trauma, fears, and pain and suffering. The jury found that the defendants did not discriminate against the child, violate the child's constitutional rights, commit assault and battery against the child, or falsely imprison the child. However, the jury did find the school board liable for negligently supervising and training three teachers in the use of restraints, which proximately caused injury and awarded the mother and child $460,000 for mental pain and suffering and the mother's lost wages.

We contacted the school district to see if any corrective actions have been taken to prevent similar incidents from occurring. According to the school's superintendent, the school district no longer uses restraints. Unrelated to the case, West Virginia also promulgated a state regulation stating that school personnel in a pre-kindergarten classroom may not restrain a child by any means other than a firm grasp around a child's arms or legs and only for as long as necessary.

According to the family's attorney, a doctor diagnosed the child with post traumatic stress disorder as a result of the restraint. Although she is now 15 years old, her mother says that she has still not returned to school and suffers anxiety when she sees a school or hears the word "teacher." In addition, she will not use public restrooms because she believes that it is wrong to urinate in public. At least one of three teachers responsible for restraining the child is still teaching in the same school.

Case 6: The four students, all males all under 6 years old, attended a special education class in a Tennessee public school, where they were assaulted and physically restrained by their teacher between early December 2003 and mid-March 2004. One of the children was diagnosed with a condition similar to Down syndrome, according to his parents.

The school had received complaints about the teacher after the 2002 to 2003 school year, prompting the Director of Special Education for the county to initiate an inquiry. As a result of these complaints, the school system developed a corrective action plan, which included installing a surveillance camera in the teacher's classroom, mentoring, and direct supervision by the school's Special Education Director.

Despite these corrective measures, the teacher's interactions with the children did not improve during the following school year. Specifically, to prevent the child from wandering, the teacher tied the child suffering from the Down syndrome type-condition to a cot with a sheet while he was wearing a 5 pound lead physical therapy vest, which was supposed to be used to help with the child's posture. The child's mother asked that school staff not restrain her son since it would be difficult to free him in the event of a fire. Despite her request, the teacher allegedly continued to restrain the boy, sometimes so tightly that a teacher's aide would spend 5 minutes or more trying to unravel the knots. In addition to the restraint there were claims that the teacher hit the children with a flyswatter, ruler, and her hand, according to a complaint filed with the Tennessee Department of Children's Services.

The Board of Education suspended the teacher in March 2004 and dismissed her in June 2004. In June 2005, a grand jury indicted the teacher on 14 counts of child abuse and 14 counts of assault. The teacher, who had no prior criminal convictions, pled guilty to one count of felony child abuse and neglect and three counts of misdemeanor assault. In February 2007, according to the terms of her plea agreement, she was placed on 3 years of probation but did not serve any jail time. According to the assistant district attorney general who handled the case, it was challenging because state law requires proof that the children were harmed, such as pictures of bruises or statements from doctors and there was no such evidence. He also said that the teacher's guilty plea and subsequent felony conviction for child abuse guaranteed that she would never be able to teach again in Tennessee. Tennessee revoked her teaching license, but we were unable to determine whether she is teaching or otherwise interacting with children in any other state.

Case 7: An 8-year-old boy was restrained by a substitute teacher who used masking tape to strap him to a chair and seal his mouth at an Illinois public school in March 2006. The child, who was diagnosed with attention-deficit hyperactivity disorder, attended a special education class with up to eight other students with various emotional or physical disabilities.

On the day of the incident, the substitute told the 8 year old and another male student in the class that they would not be allowed to play during their free time and told them to draw at their desks. In a written statement, the substitute told police that he disciplined the boys because they were "acting up and causing problems." The substitute testified that the two boys still did not remain in their seats, so he told them to sit in their chairs and put their hands behind their backs, and then he wrapped masking tape around their arms. After the boys broke free, the substitute taped them again in the same manner. The substitute testified that the students were "laughing" so he placed tape over each of their mouths and returned his attention to the class. After the 8 year old began "mumbling," the substitute removed the tape from his mouth and the child told him "his arms hurt." In a hand-written note the substitute left for the class's regular teacher, he wrote "I hope I didn't do something wrong by masking taping [the boys] to their chairs for a couple minutes. They were laughing most of the time when I did it."

The 8 year old reported the incident to his after-school daycare provider, according to the Illinois Department of Children and Family Services (DCFS). DCFS coordinated its efforts with law enforcement as well as the county's victim advocacy center and the State's Attorney Office and a grand jury ultimately charged the substitute with two felony counts of unlawful restraint and two felony counts of aggravated battery. During the trial, the school's principal testified that district policy allowed physical restraint in limited circumstances: to prevent students from harming themselves or damaging property or to remove a student who will not voluntarily leave an area. The principal also testified she did not know whether the substitute was ever given these policies.

A jury found the substitute guilty of one count of unlawful restraint and one count of aggravated battery in July 2008. The substitute was sentenced to 24 months probation, fined $1,500, perform 80 hours of community service, and undergo a psychological evaluation. The substitute still holds an Illinois state substitute teaching certificate that expires in June 2009. Prior to this incident, the substitute had been arrested in 2001 for driving under the influence of alcohol. He was sentenced to 18 months supervision and treatment for alcoholism, and fined $1,500.

Although this case was successfully prosecuted, individuals we interviewed from the State's Attorney Office and Equip for Equality (Illinois Protection and Advocacy Service) told us that seclusion and restraint cases involving children and adults with physical or mental disabilities typically have low rates of prosecution. The State's Attorney Office cited reasons such as the reluctance to further traumatize victims by having them testify, the stereotype that special needs children are unreliable witnesses, and sympathy for teachers and other staff seen as working with challenging individuals who might need to be secluded or restrained. In addition, Equip for Equality officials told us these incidents may also go underreported if children are not able to relate their experiences because they may be unable to communicate orally.

Case 8: The students were five first grade children restrained by a volunteer teacher's aide at a public elementary school in Florida in August and September 2003. The volunteer aide, who had a prior criminal record, was charged with child abuse and false imprisonment for using tape to restrain and gag her students as punishment for misbehavior.

The students, aged 6 and 7, were bound with tape in a variety of ways. The aide lashed their arms to their laps, tied their ankles together, strapped their bodies to their desks, fastened their heads to the blackboard and sealed their mouths shut. A portion of one child's hair was snatched off when the aide forcibly removed the tape. We could find no evidence to indicate that the school trained or conducted a background check on the aide, who was at the time a felon on probation for armed burglary, cocaine possession and grand theft.

After the students filed a complaint with the police, the aide surrendered and was charged with five felony counts of child abuse. She pled guilty to four counts of false imprisonment and one count of misdemeanor battery in January 2005 and was placed on 5 years probation, with the possibility of early termination of this probation after 2 and a half years and completion of all special release conditions, which included serving 75 hours of community service, taking classes in parenting and anger management, and having no contact with the students. Approximately a year later the aide was again arrested, this time for possession of cocaine and drug paraphernalia. A law enforcement officer witnessed her with a crack pipe.

Case 9: The student was a 7-year-old female enrolled in a special classroom at a public school in California when her teacher began secluding, restraining, and abusing her. The student, a small, frail girl weighing only 43 pounds, was diagnosed with Asperger's Syndrome, a form of autism characterized by language impairment and poor social skills.

According to the student's mother, the teacher secluded the girl in a walled off area in the back of the classroom accessible by only one door because she refused to do her school work. The mother alleged that when the teacher discovered that her daughter was wiggling a loose tooth, the teacher physically restrained her by making her lie face down on the floor and sitting on top of her. When the student came home from school that day, she complained to her mother, "Mommy, Mommy, my teacher hurt me, and I couldn't breathe." In June 2001, the student's mother sent a letter to the teacher instructing her to discontinue all physical restraints on her daughter. Despite these instructions, the parents alleged that restraint and other physical abuse continued. They also alleged that the girl was frequently left in seclusion for 3 hours at a time for refusing to do work. In December 2001, the parents met with the principal and the teacher and ordered the teacher to stop all physical restraints and prolonged seclusions, placing these instructions in the child's IEP.

The restraint and other mistreatment continued, according to the parents. In April 2002, the parents alleged that the teacher admitted to smearing the contents of a burrito all over the student's face and hair after she refused to eat. In July, the parents removed their daughter from the school after the teacher allegedly physically restrained her at least three times in one day during summer school. Furthermore, according to the parents' complaint, the teacher kicked the student, spun her around, and dropped her on her head. When her mother picked her up from school that day, the child had a severe abrasion to her arm, a one-inch diameter bruise on her right shoulder, and a bump on the right side of her head. The student told her mother she was "hurt all day" by her teacher. The teacher later said she restrained the student because she was a danger to herself and others. Furthermore, the teacher said the student had threatened her by waving a pair of scissors at her. According to the teacher, while she was restraining the child, her arm gave out and the student fell to the floor, injuring herself. The school's principal stated that the teacher received training once a year in applying restraints. However, this was not the first time the teacher had been accused of physically mistreating a child. Prior to the July 2002 incident, the teacher was accused of using excessive force while restraining another child in her classroom. However, the teacher did not have any prior criminal convictions.

The student's family sued the teacher, multiple school officials, and the school district. At trial, the teacher and school's principal were found liable for negligence and civil rights violations and the school district was found liable for civil rights violations. The family was initially awarded $700,000 in damages. According to the student's attorney, to avoid an appeal by the school district, the family settled with the school district and school officials. As part of the settlement agreement, though, the school district and school officials did not admit any liability. The student's family was ultimately awarded $260,000. In addition, the parties agreed to a 2- year period of judicial oversight during which the school district would be required to institute policy changes related to the discipline and behavior management of special needs children in order to achieve the goals of training, supervision, and accountability.

The school officials involved with this case are no longer employed with the school district, according to the student's attorney. However, in October 2002, the teacher began teaching in a different school district, where she remained until June 2005. She currently holds a valid California state teaching license, but we were unable to determine if she is employed as a teacher. The student is now home-schooled and living in a different state. According to the student's mother, the girl has never fully recovered from her experience.

Case 10: The student was a 9-year-old male with a learning disability who was secluded in a time out room repeatedly while enrolled in second grade in a New York public school. As part of his educational plan, his mother agreed to an IEP to assist with his learning disability. The IEP specified that the school may put the child in a 'time-out' room to correct inappropriate behavior, but only as a last resort. However, school records show that the student was placed in the time-out room regularly—75 times over a 6 month period during the 1992-1993 school year, occasionally for an hour or longer. The reasons for the confinement logged by the teachers included behaviors that were not physically aggressive; examples include, "whistling," "slouching," and "waving hands." In order to reach the room, the child was escorted out of his classroom in front of his peers, down a hallway, and to a location by the school auditorium. Although the door to the room was unlocked, a staff person would hold the door of the room closed to prevent him from leaving, and the child's hands became blistered at least once while trying to escape. On at least one occasion, the child claims he was physically restrained facedown on the floor. The school district felt that this approach was reasonable; however, a psychologist said that the child suffered from attention deficit hyperactivity disorder (ADHD), and his attorney argued that perhaps he couldn't control the behaviors that led to his confinement. As shown in pictures taken by the child's mother, the time-out room was small—approximately the length of an adult's arm span— and was lined with ripped and dirty padding. In addition, the student's mother reported that the room lacked ventilation and had an odor of "dirty feet and urine." When she visited the room and observed the conditions there, she requested that her son be transferred to another school.

The student brought a civil suit against the school district, alleging false imprisonment, negligent infliction of emotional distress, and a violation of the prohibition against unlawful seizure under the Fourth Amendment of the U.S. Constitution. The court awarded $75,000 to the student's family plus legal fees—$1,000 for each of the 75 times that the child was placed in the room. Based on our investigation, none of the educators associated with this case appear to have a criminal history. We were unable to determine whether they are still teaching.

Cases Involving Restraint from Previous Work

The following three cases from our previous work on residential treatment programs confirm the finding that face down or other restraints that block the airway can be deadly. In these cases, staff members restrained the victims by holding them face down in the ground, resulting in death by severed artery, suffocation, and abnormal heartbeat, respectively. In addition, all the teens in these cases were diagnosed with disabilities.

Case 1: The victim was a 15-year-old male who died while being restrained by two counselors. According to the victim's mother, in 2000 she enrolled her son in a wilderness program in Oregon to build his confidence and develop self-esteem in the wake of a childhood car accident. The accident had resulted in her son sustaining a severe head injury, among other injuries. According to her lawsuit, her son left the program headquarters on a group hike with three counselors and three other students. Several days into the multiday hike, the victim refused to return to the campsite after being escorted by a counselor about 200 yards to relieve himself. Two counselors then attempted to lead him back to the campsite. According to an account of the incident, when he continued to refuse, they tried to force him to return and they all fell to the ground together. The two counselors subsequently held the victim face down in the dirt until he stopped struggling; by one account a counselor sat on the victim for almost 45 minutes. When the counselors realized the victim was no longer breathing, they telephoned for help and requested a 911 operator's advice on administering CPR. While the mother was driving to the hospital, her son's doctor called, advised her to pull to the side of the road, and informed her that her son had died. The victim's mother told us that she was informed, after the autopsy, that the main artery in her son's neck had been torn. The cause of death was listed as a homicide.

In September 2000, after the boy's death, one of the counselors was charged with criminally negligent homicide. A grand jury subsequently declined to indict him.

In early 2001, the mother of the victim filed a $1.5 million wrongful death lawsuit against the program, its parent company, and its president. The lawsuit was settled in 2002 for an undisclosed amount.

Table 2. Summary of Cases from Previous Work on Residential Treatment Centers for Troubled Youth

Case	Victim information	Program attended	Date of death	Case details related to use of restraint
1	Male, 15, Oregon resident	Oregon wilderness therapy program	2000	Refused to return to campsite but did not behave violently. Restrained by staff and held face down to the groundfor almost 45 minutes. Died of severed artery in neck.
2	Male, 12, Texas resident	Texas residential treatment center	2005	Victim was angry and started banging his head against the ground. A 5 feet,10 inch, muscular staff member placed the 87-pound victim into a facedown restraint. Several witnesses claimed they saw the staff member lying across the back of the victim. Victim complained he couldn't breathe and eventually became unresponsive, at which point the staff member removed the restraint. Attempts to revive victim failed.
3	Male, 16, Pennsylvania resident	Pennsylvania psychiatric residential treatment center	2006	Victim was placed under "intense observation" for attempting to run away from the program. Victim was ordered to put the hood of his sweatshirt down so that staff could see his face, but victim refused. Three staff members brought the victim to another room and placed him in facedown restraint. After 10 minutes of the restraint, victim complained that he couldn't breathe. Victim died at the hospital 3 hours later from an abnormal heartbeat.

Sources: Records including police reports, court documents, and interviews.

Case 2: The victim, who died in 2005, was a 12-year-old male. Documents obtained from the Texas Department of Family and Protective Services indicate that the victim had a troubled family background. He was taken into state care along with his siblings at the age of 6. As a ward of the state, the victim spent several years in various foster placements and youth programs before being placed in a private residential treatment center in August 2005. The program advertised itself as a "unique facility" that specialized in services for boys with learning disabilities and behavioral or emotional issues. The victim's caretakers chose to place him in this program because he was emotionally disturbed. Records indicate that he was covered by Medicaid.

On the evening of his death, the victim refused to take a shower and was ordered to sit on an outside porch. According to police reports, the victim began to bang his head repeatedly against the concrete floor of the porch, leading a staff member to drag him away from the porch and place him in a "lying basket restraint" for his own protection. During this restraint, the 4 feet 91/2 inch tall, 87-pound boy was forced to lie on his stomach with his arms crossed under him as the staff member, a muscular male 5 feet 10 inches tall, held him still. Some of the children who witnessed the restraint said they saw the staff member lying across the victim's back. During the restraint, the victim fought against the staff member and yelled at him to stop. The staff member told police that the victim complained that he could not breathe, but added that children "always say that they cannot breathe during a restraint." According to police reports, after about 10 minutes of forced restraint, the staff member observed that the victim had calmed down and was no longer fighting back. The staff member slowly released the restraint and asked the victim if he wanted a jacket. The victim did not respond. The staff member told police he interpreted the victim's silence as an unwillingness to talk because of anger about the restraint. He said he waited for a minute while the victim lay silently on the ground. When the victim did not respond to his question a second time, he tapped the victim on the shoulder and rolled him over. The staff member observed that the victim was pale and could not detect a pulse. All efforts to revive the victim failed, and he was declared dead at a nearby hospital.

Although the Texas Department of Family and Protective Services alleged that the victim's death was because of physical abuse, the official certificate of death stated that it was an accident and a grand jury declined to press charges against the staff member performing the restraint. However, the victim's siblings obtained a civil settlement against the program and the staff member for an undisclosed amount.

Case 3: The victim was 16 years old when he died, in February 2006, at a private psychiatric residential treatment facility in Pennsylvania for boys with behavioral or emotional problems. He was a large boy—6 feet 1 inch in height and weighing about 250 pounds—and suffered from bipolar disorder and asthma. The cost for placement in this facility was primarily paid for by Medicaid.

According to state investigative documents we obtained, the victim was placed in intensive observation after he attempted to run away. As part of the intensive observation, he was forced to sit in a chair in the hallway of the facility and was restricted from participating in some activities with other residents. On the day of his death, staff allowed the victim to participate in arts, crafts, and games with the other youth, but would not let him leave the living area to attend other recreational activities. Instead, staff told the victim that he would have to return to his chair in the hallway. In addition, staff told him that he would have to move his chair so that he could not see the television in another room. The victim complied, moving his chair out of view of the television, but put up the hood of his sweatshirt and turned his back toward the staff. The staff ordered him to take down his hood, but he refused. When one of the staff walked up to him and pulled his hood down, the victim jumped out of his chair and made a threatening posture with his fists, saying he did not want to be touched. The staff member and two coworkers then brought the victim to another room and held him facedown on the floor with his arms pulled up behind his back. The victim struggled against the restraint, yelling and trying to kick the three staff members holding him down. After about 10 minutes, the victim became limp and started breathing heavily. He complained that he was having difficulties breathing. One staff member unzipped his sweatshirt and loosened the collar of his shirt, but rather than improve, the victim became unresponsive. The staff called emergency services and began CPR. The victim was taken by ambulance to a hospital, where he died a little more than 3 hours later. In the victim's autopsy report his death was ruled accidental, as caused by asphyxia and an abnormal heartbeat (cardiac dysrhythmia).

No criminal charges were filed in regard to the victim's death. The victim's mother filed a civil suit over her son's death against the facility. The suit was pending at the time we completed our investigation.

Mr. Chairman and Members of the Committee, this concludes my statement. I would be pleased to answer any questions that you or other members of the committee may have at this time.

Appendix I: Summary of State Laws Related to the Use of Restraints and Seclusions in Public and Private Schools

The following list provides an overview of laws related to the use of restraints or seclusions in public and private schools in all 50 states and the District of Columbia.

Alabama

Ala. Code § 16-1-14 (Education; General Provisions)

- Local school boards may prescribe rules and regulations, subject to State Board of Education approval, that isolate or separate pupils who create disciplinary problems in any classroom or other school activity and whose presence in the class may be detrimental to the best interest and welfare of the class as a whole.

Alaska

Alaska admin. Code tit. 4, §§ 07.010 - .900 (Education and Early Development; Student Rights and Responsibilities)

- The use of corporal punishment in Alaska public schools is prohibited. However, the definition of corporal punishment does not include the use of reasonable and necessary physical restraint of a student to protect the student or others from physical injury, to obtain possession of a weapon or other dangerous object from a student, to maintain reasonable order in the classroom or on school grounds, or to protect property from serious damage or destruction.

Arizona

None

Arkansas

005-18 Ark. Code R. § 020 (Department of Education; Special Education and Related Services)

- Public agencies that provide education to children with disabilities must follow standards for use of a time-out seclusion room. Time-out seclusion should be used only for behaviors that are destructive to property, aggressive toward others, or severely disruptive to the class environment. Also, it should only be used as a last resort when less restrictive means are ineffective. Only necessary reasonable force may be used to place a student in such a room and, in general, time-out is not an appropriate intervention for classroom use with any students older than 12 unless they have made a contractual agreement for its use. Rooms must meet certain guidelines, such as minimum size restrictions, and provide for continuous visual and auditory monitoring. The door should be such that it cannot be locked. The use of seclusion time-out must be stated in the student's IEP and have parental consent with documented written procedures. Maximum time to be spent in the room varies from 5 to 20 minutes, depending on the grade level. Careful consideration must be taken in extending the prescribed length of the seclusion. Records must be kept of each use of the room. Personnel must be adequately trained and supervised.

California

Cal. Code Regs. tit. 5, § 3052 (Education; California Department Of Education; Handicapped Children; Special Education; Implementation)

- Emergency interventions for special education students may only be used to control unpredictable, spontaneous behavior which poses a clear and present danger of serious physical harm to the individual or others and which cannot be immediately prevented by a response less restrictive than the temporary application of a technique used to contain the behavior.
- Emergency interventions may not include locked seclusion, the use of force that exceeds that which is reasonable and necessary under the

circumstances, or the employment of a device or material or object which simultaneously immobilize all four extremities, except that techniques such as prone containment may be used as an emergency intervention by staff trained in such a procedure.

- Parents must be notified within one school day whenever an emergency intervention is used, and a Behavioral Emergency Report must be completed that includes details of the incident. The number of reports created annually is reported to the state Department of Education.
- No intervention may be used which is designed or likely to cause physical pain; which denies adequate sleep, food, water; shelter, bedding, physical comfort, or access to bathroom facilities; that precludes adequate supervision of the individual; or which deprives the individual of one or more of his or her senses.

Colorado

Colo. Rev. Stat. §§ 26-20-101 to -109 (Human Services Code; Protection of persons from restraint)

- Certain state agencies, including the Colorado Department of Education, are subject to restrictions on the use of restraints. These include the requirement that restraints may only be used in cases of emergency and after the failure of less restrictive alternatives, unless such alternatives would be inappropriate or ineffective under the circumstances. Restraints may only be used for the purpose of preventing the continuation or renewal of an emergency, for the time period necessary, and with no more force than is necessary. However, the term "restraint" does not include the holding of an individual for less than 5 minutes by a staff person for the protection of the individual or other persons.
- Physical restraints must not place excess pressure on the chest or back or impede the ability to breathe, and staff must check to ensure that the breathing of the individual is not compromised.
- Agencies shall ensure that staff utilizing restraint are trained in its appropriate use, and agencies shall ensure each use of restraint is appropriately documented.

- Additional restrictions apply to the use of mechanical or chemical restraints.

1 Colo. Code Regs. § 301-45 (Department of education; Colorado State Board of Education; Protection of persons from restraint)

- Restraints shall only be used in an emergency and with extreme caution and are limited to situations in which there is serious, probable, and imminent threat of bodily harm. In addition to formally adopting the above statutes, the regulations specify that restraints must never be used as a form of discipline or as a threat to control or gain compliance of a student's behavior. Only trained staff may administer restraints, and restraints may not be used in such a way that the student is prevented from breathing or communicating. A restrained student must be continuously monitored to ensure breathing is not compromised, and a student shall be released within 15 minutes, except where precluded for safety reasons. When the restraint is no longer necessary to protect the student or the safety others, it must be removed. A student's behavior plan must address the specific circumstances, procedures, and staff involved if there is a possibility that restraint may be used as part of crisis management. When it is anticipated that restraint will be used in an emergency situation, written parental permission must be obtained. Staff training must include a continuum of prevention and de-escalation techniques, as well as techniques that allow restraint in an upright or sitting position. If a restraint is used, a written report must be submitted within one school day detailing the incident, the parents must be notified as soon as possible, and the incident must go through a review process.

Connecticut

Conn. Gen. Stat. §§ 46a-150 to -154 (Human Rights; Physical Restraint, Medication and Seclusion of Persons Receiving Care, Education, or Supervision in a School, Institution, or facility)

- Providers of education to special education students may not use life-threatening physical restraints, defined as those restraints that restrict the flow of air into a person's lungs, whether by chest compression or other means. Involuntary physical restraint may not be used on special education students except as emergency intervention designed to prevent immediate or imminent injury to the person at risk or to others. The restraint may not be used for discipline or convenience and is not as a substitute for a less restrictive alternative. The use of physical restraint must be documented in the student's record, and parents must be notified. A special education student who is physically restrained must be continually monitored by a provider or assistant and regularly evaluated for indications of physical distress. Each incident must be fully documented, and all providers and assistant providers must be trained in the use of physical restraint, including de-escalation techniques, prevention strategies, types of physical restraints, differences between life-threatening restraints and other types, differences between permissible restraints and pain compliance techniques, and more. Incidents must be compiled and reported annually to the state.

- Special education students may not be placed in seclusion except as an emergency intervention to prevent immediate or imminent injury to the person or to others. The seclusion may not be used for discipline or convenience and is not used as a substitute for a less restrictive alternative. The use of seclusion must be documented in the student's record, and parents must be notified. A special education student who is involuntarily placed in seclusion must be frequently monitored by a provider or assistant and regularly evaluated for indications of physical distress. Each incident must be fully documented, and all providers and assistant providers must be trained in the use of seclusions. Incidents must be compiled and reported annually to the state.

Delaware

14-900 Del. Code Regs. § 929 (Department of Education; Special Populations)

- While "restraint" or "seclusion" are not discussed directly, a school's "emergency intervention procedures" and "behavior management procedures" for children with autism must be reviewed by the state's

Human Rights Committee and Peer Review Committee. Parents must give informed consent for the use of each behavior management procedure, and may withdraw that consent at any time.

District of Columbia

D.c. Code §§ 38-2561.01 - .16 (Educational Institutions; Special Education; Nonpublic Schools)

- "Aversive intervention" includes a variety of practices, including the use of chemical restraints; withholding adequate sleep, shelter, clothing, bedding, or bathroom facilities; and withholding meals, essential nutrition, or hydration. Except in certain limited circumstances, no student whose education is funded by the D.C. government may be placed in a nonpublic special education school or program that allows the use of these aversive interventions.

Florida

None.

Georgia

None.

Hawaii

Hawaii Rev. Stat. § 302a-1 141 (Government; Education; Education; Provisions Affecting System Structure; Organization)

- No physical punishment of any kind may be inflicted upon any pupil, but reasonable force may be used by a teacher in order to restrain a pupil in attendance at school from hurting oneself or any other person or property.

Idaho

None.

Illinois

105 Ill. Comp. Stat. 5/2-3. 130 (Schools; Common Schools; School Code; State Board of Education – Powers and Duties)

- The State Board of Education is required to promulgate rules governing the use of time out and physical restraint in public schools.

105 Ill. comp. stat. 5/10-20.33 (Schools; Common Schools; School Code; School Boards)

- Until rules are adopted by the State Board of Education, the use of physical restraints is prohibited except where the student poses a physical risk to persons, there is no medical contraindication to its use, and the staff applying it have been trained in its safe application. "Restraint" does not include momentary periods of physical restriction by direct person-to-person contact with limited force that is designed to prevent a student from completing an act that would result in potential physical harm to persons or damage to property, or to remove a student who is unwilling to leave an area voluntarily. Uses of restraint must be documented and parents notified.
- Until rules are adopted by the State Board of Education, timeout rooms cannot lock other than with a mechanism that engages when a key or handle is being held by a person, cannot be a confining space such as a closet or box, and cannot be a room where the student cannot be continually observed.

Ll. Admin. Code tit. 28, §§ 1.280, .285 (education and cultural resources; education; State board of education; Public school recognition; Public schools evaluation, Recognition and supervision; School governance)

- The restrictions listed in 105 Ill. Comp. Stat. 5/10-20.33 are repeated and adopted. In addition, physical restraint may only be used as a means of maintaining discipline and only to the extent necessary to preserve the safety of students and others. It may not be used as a form of punishment. Only specific, planned techniques are permitted.

- Students are not subject to restraint for using profanity, verbal displays of disrespect, or verbal threats unless accompanied by a means or intent to carry out the threat. Except under certain limited circumstances, the use of mechanical or chemical restraints is prohibited. Use of restraint shall take into consideration the safety and security of the student, and it shall not rely on pain as an intentional method of control. If the student uses sign language or an augmentative mode of primary communication, the student shall be permitted to have the student's hands free of restraint for brief periods, unless the adult determines that such freedom appears likely to result in harm to self or others. The restraint must end as soon as the student is no longer in imminent danger of causing physical harm to persons.
- Detailed records of each incident must be kept, and parents must be notified within 24 hours. Training must include alternatives to restraint, de-escalation procedures, the experience of administering and receiving a variety of restraint techniques, how to monitor for physical signs of distress, and retraining every 2 years. School districts must review the use of restraints annually.
- Isolated time out may only be used as a means of maintaining discipline and only to the extent necessary to preserve the safety of students and others. It may not be used as a form of punishment.
- Enclosures used for isolated time out must meet size requirements, be free of materials that can be used to cause harm, and be designed to permit continuous visual monitoring of and communication with the student. Doors, if used, must be steel or wood with a solid-core constriction, with an unbreakable viewing panel. An adult must remain within two feet and must be able to see the student at all times. If the enclosure has a locking mechanism, it must only be engaged when it is held in position by a person, or if electronically engaged, must automatically release if the building's fire alarm system is activated. A student may not be kept in isolated time out for more than 30 minutes after the problematic behavior has ceased.
- Detailed records of each incident must be kept, and parents must be notified within 24 hours. School districts must review the use of isolated time out annually.

Ill. Admin. Code tit. 23, § 401.250 (Education and Cultural Resources; education; State Board of education; Nonpublic Elementary and Secondary Schools; Special Education Facilities under Section 14-7.02 of the School Code; Operations Requirements)

- Private, special education facilities must have their staff trained in the use of isolated time out and restraint according to the requirements of Ill. Admin. Code tit. 28, §§ 1.280, .285

Indiana

None.

Iowa

Iowa Admin. Code §§ 281-103.1 - .8 (Education Department; Protection of Children; Corporal Punishment Ban; Restraint; Physical Confinement and Detention)

- Corporal punishment is prohibited, but does not include using reasonable and necessary force: in order to quell a disturbance or prevent physical harm to any person; in order to obtain possession of a weapon or other dangerous object; for the purposes of self-defense or defense of others; for the protection of property; to remove a disruptive pupil from class or school premises, or from school-sponsored activities off school premises; to prevent a student from the self- infliction of harm; or to protect the safety of others.
- Physical restraint shall not be used as discipline for minor infractions and may be used only after other disciplinary techniques have been attempted, if reasonable. All school employees must receive adequate and periodic training, which must include alternatives to restraint, crisis prevention and intervention, de-escalation techniques, and its safe and effective use. The restraint must be reasonable and necessary in duration, and each occurrence must be documented. Parents must be notified of any occurrence the same day, if possible.

- Prone restraints are prohibited, as is any restraint that obstructs the airway of any child. If the student uses sign language or an augmentative mode of primary communication, the student must be permitted to have the student's hands free of restraint for brief periods, unless an employee determines that such freedom appears likely to result in harm to self or others.
- Physical confinement shall not be used as discipline for minor infractions and may be used only after other disciplinary techniques have been attempted, if reasonable under the circumstances. All school employees must receive adequate and periodic training, which must include alternatives to seclusion, and the safe and effective use of physical confinement. Parents must be notified of any occurrence the same day, if possible.
- If a student is physically confined, the area of confinement must be of reasonable dimensions, and must be free from hazards and dangerous objects or instruments, considering the characteristics and condition of the student. There must be sufficient light and ventilation, a comfortable temperature, and reasonable break periods to attend to bodily needs. The time period must be reasonable considering the characteristics and condition of the student, and continuous adult supervision is required. If the room has a locking mechanism, it must only be engaged when it is held in position by a person, or if electronically engaged, must automatically release if the building's fire alarm system is activated or electrical power is interrupted.

Kansas

None.

Kentucky

None.

Louisiana

None.

Maine

Me. Rev. Stat. Ann. Tit. 20, § 4502 (Education; elementary and Secondary Education; Elementary and Secondary Schools; Basic School Approval)

- Timeout areas must be well ventilated, sufficiently lighted, and may not be locked. The student must be either supervised by staff in the room or observed and heard by a person outside the room.

05-071-033 Me. Code R. §§ 1.1 – 5.1 (Department of Education; General; Regulations Governing Time Out Rooms, Therapeutic Restraints, and Aversives in Public Schools and Approved Private Schools

- Local school administrative units and approved private schools must develop policies for isolated timeout rooms and therapeutic restraint consistent with these regulations. Policies must be reviewed at least annually. Each use shall be documented, and parents must be notified as soon practical.
- Therapeutic restraint may be used by trained staff to prevent injury to the student or others. It may be used either as an emergency intervention or as part of an intervention plan, but only after less intrusive efforts have been attempted. The restraint shall use the least amount of physical contact necessary, and requires the presence of at least two adults, unless there is an emergency situation. Restraint shall not exceed one hour, unless the student is still presenting dangerous behavior. Mechanical and chemical restraints are prohibited. Individuals must be trained in the use of restraints, including de-escalation techniques.
- Timeout rooms are used to reduce dangerous behavior and only after less intrusive interventions have failed. They may be used either as an

emergency intervention or as part of an intervention plan, but not for punitive purposes, staff convenience, or to control minor misbehavior.

- Use of the room shall not exceed one hour, unless the student is still presenting dangerous behavior. Students in a timeout room shall be directly observed at all times. Rooms must meet certain physical requirement, and have adequate light, hear, and ventilation. The door may not be locked, and must include an unbreakable observation window.

Maryland

Md. Code regs. 13a.08.04.01 - .06 (State Board of Education; Students; Student Behavior Interventions)

- The restraint, exclusion and seclusion policies apply to public agencies and nonpublic schools. Restraint and seclusion may only be used: after less restrictive approaches have been considered; in a humane, safe, and effective manner; without intent to harm or create undue discomfort; and consistent with medical and psychological limitations and the student's intervention plan. Schools must review these policies annually.
- Restraint does not include briefly holding a student to calm, comfort, or escort the student safely, moving a disruptive student who is unwilling to leave the area if other methods are unsuccessful, or intervening in a fight. The use of restraint is prohibited unless there is an emergency and the restraint is necessary to protect persons from imminent, serious, physical harm; it is permitted under the student's IEP; or the parents of a nondisabled student have provided written consent while a behavior plan is being developed. Only trained school personnel may apply restraints, and they may only use reasonable force. The use of mechanical restraints is prohibited except in specific circumstances. Each instance of restraint must be documented, and parents must be notified within 24 hours.
- "Exclusion" means removing a student to a supervised area for a limited period of time. This may be used when the student's behavior unreasonably interferes with the student's or other's learning, or the behavior is an emergency and the exclusion is necessary to protect

persons from imminent, serious, physical harm. School personnel must be able to see the student at all time, the exclusion area must provide adequate lighting, ventilation, and furniture, and the area must be unlocked and free of barriers. Exclusion periods may not exceed 30 minutes.

- "Seclusion" means the confinement of a student alone in a room from which the student is physically prevented from leaving. The use of seclusion is prohibited, unless there is an emergency and the seclusion is necessary to protect persons from imminent, serious, physical harm; it is permitted under the student's IEP; or the parents of a nondiabled student have provided written consent while a behavior plan is being developed. Seclusion rooms must be free of objects that could cause harm, provide an adequate view of the student, and provide adequate lighting and ventilation. School personnel must view the student at all times, and reassess every 30 minutes. Each instance of seclusion must be documented, and parents must be notified within 24 hours.

Massachusetts

603 Mass. Code Regs. 18.05 (Department of Education; Program and Safety Standards for Approved Public or Private Day and Residential Special Education School Programs)

- Schools providing special education services must provide to parents, prior to admission, a copy of the school's policies and procedure related to restraints, exclusion, time out, and other aversive procedures. Written informed consent from the parent is required prior to utilizing these techniques.
- Day special educational programs, residential special education programs, and special education programs within mental health facilities must all comply with their respective regulations regarding the use of restraints and seclusion.
- A school's behavior management policy regarding seclusion must include guidelines for staff, the duration of the procedure including higher approval needed for any period longer than 30 minutes, the requirement that students shall be observable at all times, a procedure for staff to directly observe the student every 15 minutes,

documentation requirements, and the requirements that the room may not be locked and must be safe.

603 Mass. Code Regs. 46.01 - .07 (Department of Education; Physical Restraint)

- This regulation applies only to students in publicly funded elementary and secondary education programs. Physical restraints may only be used in emergency situations, after less intrusive alternatives have failed, and with extreme caution. Schools must develop written procedures that are reviewed annually and include an explanation of the method of restraint, training requirements, reporting requirements, and complaint procedures.
- All staff must be trained within the first month of each school year on types of restraints with related safety considerations, and some staff must receive additional in-depth training that includes de-escalation procedures, methods for evaluating the risk of harm in individual situations, the simulated experience of administering and receiving restraint, and more.
- Restraint may only be used when non-physical interventions would not be effective, and the student's behavior poses a threat of imminent, serious, physical harm to self or others. Only reasonable force may be used. Restraint may not be used as a means of punishment or as a response to property destruction, disruption of school order, refusal to comply with school rules or directives, or verbal threats that do not constitute a threat of imminent, serious, physical harm. Only trained personnel may administer restraints, except to protect persons from imminent, serious physical harm, and when possible the restraint must be witnessed by at least one other adult. The safest method available and appropriate must be used, and floor or prone restraints are prohibited unless the method is required and the staff member has received in-depth training. Restraint must be discontinued as soon as possible; if it continues for more than 20 minutes, additional reporting requirements apply. No restraint may be administered in such a way that the student is prevented from breathing or speaking, and staff must continuously monitor the physical status of the student. Each incident must be reviewed and documented, and restraint reports may be reviewed by the Department of Education. Parents must be notified as soon as possible.

Michigan

Mich. Comp. Laws serv. § 380.1312 (School Code of 1976; the Revised School Code; Boards of Education, Powers and Duties Generally)

- Corporal punishment is prohibited. However, school personnel may use reasonable physical force: upon a pupil to restrain or remove a pupil whose behavior is interfering with the orderly exercise and performance of school district or public school academy functions, if that pupil has refused to comply with a request to refrain from further disruptive acts; for self-defense or the defense of another person; to prevent self-injury; to quell a disturbance that threatens physical injury to any person; to obtain possession of a weapon or other dangerous object upon or within the control of a pupil; or, to protect property.

Minnesota

Minn. Stat. §§ 121a.58 -.67 (Education Code: Prekindergarten – Grade 12; Student Rights, Responsibilities, and Behavior; Discipline, all Students)

- Corporal punishment is not allowed. However, a teacher or principal may use reasonable force when necessary to correct or restrain a student or prevent bodily harm or death.
- The Commissioner of the Minnesota Department of Education must promulgate rules that govern the use of aversive procedures on children with a disability. These rules must require that the planned application of aversive and deprivation procedures only be instituted after developing a behavior intervention plan, and that education personnel will notify parents on the same day that aversive or deprivation procedures are used.
- Rules for the use of aversive procedures on children with a disability must also include requirements: that the use of locked time-out have standards such as requiring a safe environment, continuous monitoring, ventilation, adequate space, a locking mechanism that disengages automatically when not continuously engaged, and more;

that the commissioner make unannounced on-site visits to monitor locked time- out rooms; and that a student may only be placed in locked time-out if it is part of the student's behavior intervention plan, or it is an emergency and only for the emergency's duration.

Minn. R. 3525.2900 (Department of Education; Children with a Disability)

- In addition to adopting the above restrictions, students in time-out seclusion must have adequate access to drinking water and a bathroom for a time-out that exceeds 15 minutes. Documentation of the time-out is required. The time-out area must be a safe environment without hazards; have adequate light, heat, and ventilation; have an observation window; and meet size specifications that allow the pupil to stand, stretch arms, and lie down.

Mississippi

None.

Missouri

None.

Montana

Mont. Code ann. § 20-4-302 (Education; Teacher, Superintendents, and Principals; Teachers' Powers, Duties, and Privileges)

- Corporal punishment is prohibited. However, school personnel may use physical restraint that is reasonable and necessary, even if it causes physical pain, to quell a disturbance, provide self-protection, protect persons from physical injury, obtain possession of a weapon or dangerous object from the pupil, maintain the orderly conduct of a pupil, or protect property from serious harm.

Mont. Admin. R. 10.16.3346 (Department of Education; Special Education; Services)

- "Aversive treatment procedures" include physical restraint and isolation time-out. Aversive treatment procedures may be used on a special education student who exhibits behaviors which pose a risk of physical harm to the student or others, a risk of significant damage to property, or significantly disruptive or dangerous behaviors. Aversive treatment procedures must be designed to address the behavioral needs of an individual student, be approved by the IEP team, and may not be used as punishment, for the convenience of staff, or as a substitute for positive behavioral interventions. Any procedure intended solely to cause pain is prohibited.
- Mechanical restraints are prohibited, except in limited circumstances.
- A student in isolation time out must be under direct constant visual observation of a staff person. Isolation in a locked room is prohibited.

Nebraska

None.

Nevada

Nev. Rev. Stat. Ann. §§ 388.521 - .5315 (Education; System of Public Instruction; Pupils with Disabilities and Gifted and Talented Pupils; Use of Aversive Intervention, Physical Restraint and Mechanical Restraint on Pupils with Disabilities)

- Mechanical restraints are prohibited, unless under certain circumstances where a medical order authorizing its use has been obtained. Additional rules also apply to the use of mechanical restraints.
- Physical restraints may not be used on a pupil with a disability, unless an emergency exists where the restraint is necessary to protect the physical safety of persons from an immediate threat of physical injury or to protect against an immediate threat of severe property damage.

The restraint may be for no longer than is necessary, and the use of force may not exceed that which is reasonable and necessary under the circumstances. Instances must be documented and reported to the school district and the parents. Staff authorized to carry out physical restraints must be trained in its use.

- "Aversive intervention" includes the placement of a person in a room, alone, where release from the room is prohibited. Aversive interventions are prohibited when used on a pupil with a disability.

New Hampshire

N.H. Code Admin. R. Ann. Ed. 1113.04 - .09 (Board of Education; Standards for the Education of Children with Disabilities; Requirements for the Development and Operation of Programs for Children with Disabilities Administered by Local Education Agencies)

- Public or private providers of special education may not employ aversive behavioral interventions, except in response to the threat of imminent, serious physical harm. These include any procedure intended to cause physical pain, placement of a child in an unsupervised or unobserved room from which the child can not exit, and physical restraint. However, if authorized in writing by a physician and an IEP team, then non-medical mechanical restraint and physical restraint not in response to imminent, serious, physical harm may be used. Staff must be trained to use procedures and in alternative de- escalation techniques, and the parents must give informed consent for the use of these procedures separate from the IEP consent.

New Jersey

None.

New Mexico

N.M. Stat. Ann. §§ 32a-6a-1 to -10 (Children's Code; Children's Mental Health and Developmental Disabilities Act)

- "Aversive interventions," which includes interventions causing physical pain and isolation, are prohibited. When providing treatment or habilitation services to children with severe developmental disabilities, physical restraint and seclusion may not be used except in an emergency situation in which it's necessary to protect a child or another from imminent, serious physical harm or unless a less intrusive intervention has failed. Programs shall provide a copy of the restraint and seclusion polices and procedures to the child's legal custodian. Staff administering restraints and seclusions must be trained in positive behavior interventions, methods for identifying and defusing potentially dangerous behavior, and restraint and seclusion. Incidents of restraint and seclusion must be documented, and the child's legal custodian must be notified immediately. After the incident, there must be a debriefing with the child.
- Only reasonable force as is necessary to protect the child or other person from imminent and serious physical harm may be used. The restraint must be reassessed at least every 30 minutes. Mechanical restraints are prohibited except under certain circumstances.
- Seclusion may only be applied by trained staff, and the seclusion room must be free of hazards, provide staff an adequate and continuous view of the child, and provide adequate lighting and ventilation. Staff must view the child at all times, and must reassess at least every 30 minutes.

New York

N.Y. Comp. Codes r. & regs. Tit. 8, § 19.5 (Education Department; Rules of the Board of Regents; Education Practices)

- Corporal punishment is prohibited. However, reasonable force may be used to protect oneself or any person from physical injury, to protect property, or to restrain or remove a pupil whose behavior is interfering with the orderly exercise and performance of school functions, powers and duties.

- Aversive interventions, defined as interventions intended to induce pain or discomfort for the purpose of eliminating maladaptive behaviors, are prohibited. This includes movement limitations used as a punishment.

N.Y. Comp. Codes r. & regs. Tit. 8, § 200.22 (Education Department; Regulations of the Commissioner; Handicapped Children; Children with Handicapping Conditions)

- A behavioral intervention plan shall not include the use of aversive interventions, but a child-specific exception may be granted under certain circumstances where the student is displaying aggressive behaviors that threaten the physical well being of the student or others. The use of aversive interventions may only be done by trained staff and with parental consent.
- Emergency interventions involving the use of reasonable physical force is permissible in situations in which alternative procedures cannot be reasonably employed. They may not be used as punishment, and staff must be provided with appropriate training in safe and effective restraint procedures. Each incident must be documented, and parents must be notified.
- Time out rooms are only to be used in conjunction with a behavioral intervention plan, except for unanticipated situations that pose an immediate concern for physical safety. A student may not be placed in a locked room or in a room where the student cannot be continuously observed and supervised. The room must be adequate size to allow the student to move about and recline, it should be without hazards, and have adequate lighting, ventilation, and temperature. The room must be unlocked and the door able to be opened from the inside.
- Schools must develop policies that include factors that precipitate the use of the room, time limitations, staff training, data collection, and information to be provided to parents. Staff must continuously monitor the student. A student's IEP must specify the use of a time out room, and parents must be given the opportunity to see the physical space and receive a copy of the school's policy.

North Carolina

N.C. Gen. Stat. § 115c-391.1 (Elementary and Secondary Education; Students; Discipline)

- School personnel must notify the principal of any use of aversive procedures, any use of physical restraint resulting in observable physical injury to a student, or any use of seclusion that exceeds 10 minutes or the time specified in the behavior intervention plan. The student's parents must be promptly notified, and the incident must be documented.
- Physical restraint is prohibited, except as reasonably needed to obtain possession of a weapon or other dangerous object, to maintain order or prevent or break up a fight, for self-defense, to ensure the safety of any person, to prevent imminent destruction of property, or if used as provided for in a student's IEP. Physical restraint is not permitted when used solely as a disciplinary consequence.
- Mechanical restraint is prohibited, except under certain circumstances.
- Seclusion is the confinement of a student alone in an enclosed space from which the student is physically prevented from leaving by locking hardware or other means. Seclusion is prohibited, except as reasonably needed to respond to a person in control of a weapon or other dangerous object, to maintain order or prevent or break up a fight, for self-defense, to respond to a student's behavior which poses a threat of imminent physical harm to self or others or imminent substantial destruction of property, or when used as specified in the student's IEP.
- The student in seclusion must be monitored by an adult who is able to see and hear the student at all times, and the seclusion must be released upon cessation of the behaviors that led to the seclusion. The seclusion space must have been approved by the local education agency and have appropriate light, ventilation, and temperature, and be free of hazards. Seclusion is not permitted when used solely as a disciplinary consequence.
- Isolation is a behavior management technique in which a student is placed alone in an enclosed space from which the student is not prevented from leaving. Isolation is permitted provided that the space used has appropriate light, ventilation, and temperature; the duration

is reasonable in light of the purpose; the student is reasonable monitored; and, the space is free of hazards.

North Dakota

None.

Ohio

Ohio Rev. Code ann. § 3319.41 (Education – Libraries; Schools – Superintendent, Teachers, Employees; School Reports)

- Corporal punishment is prohibited, unless the board of education of a school district has taken certain steps to permit it. However, staff may use and apply such amount of force and restraint as is reasonable and necessary to quell a disturbance threatening physical injury to others, to obtain possession of weapons or other dangerous objects upon the person or within the control of the pupil, for the purpose of self-defense, or for the protection of persons or property.

Oklahoma

None.

Oregon

Or. Admin. R. 581-021-0060 to -0062 (Oregon Department of Education; School Governance and Student Conduct; Student Conduct and DIScipline)

- Corporal punishment is prohibited. However, corporal punishment does not include physical pain or discomfort resulting from physical restraint or seclusion that is part of a behavior support plan, that includes an individual limit on the number of incidents within a specified time period, and that is carried out under set policies and procedures.

- The use of physical restraint or seclusion may only be used as part of a behavior support plan that was developed with the parents, when less restrictive interventions would not be effective and the student's behavior poses a threat of imminent, serious, physical harm to the student or others; or, in an emergency as necessary to maintain order or to prevent a student from harming him/herself, other students, and school staff or property.
- Restraint or seclusion may only be used for as long as the behavior poses a threat of imminent, serious physical harm. Staff must continuously monitor a student's status during the restraint or seclusion. Staff must be trained to use restraint or seclusion, including training in prevention and de-escalation techniques. Parental notification by the end of the day is required, and each incident must be documented.
- Seclusion rooms must allow for a full view of the student at all times, and be free of potentially hazardous conditions.

Pennsylvania

22 Pa. Code § 14.133 (Education; State Board of Education; Miscellaneous Provisions; Special Education Services and Programs; IEP)

- Restraints to control acute or episodic aggressive or self-injurious behavior may only be used when the student is a clear and present danger to himself, other students, or employees, and only when less restrictive techniques are less effective. Parental notification is required. The use of restraints may only be included in an IEP when: the restraint is utilized with specific component elements of positive behavior support; the restraint is used in conjunction with the teaching of alternate behavior; staff are authorized to use the procedure and have receiving required training; and there is a plan for eliminating the use of restraint through the application of positive behavior support. Parental consent must be obtained prior to the use of restraints. The use of prone restraints is prohibited. Data on the use of restraints must be maintained and reported. Restraint may not be used for the convenience of staff or as punishment. Mechanical restraints may only be used in certain circumstances.

- Locked rooms, locked boxes or other structures or spaces from which the student cannot readily exit are prohibited.

Rhode Island

08-010-013 R.I. Code R. §§ 1.0 – 10.0 (Department of Elementary and Secondary Education; Board of Regents for Elementary and Secondary Education; Physical Restraint)

- Public education programs must develop procedures regarding the use of physical restraint and crisis intervention. These must be reviewed annually and made available to parents. Staff must receive annual training on the restraint policy, de-escalation techniques, types of restraints and related safety considerations, and how to administer restraint in accordance with known medical or psychological limitations applicable to an individual student. Some staff must receive advanced training, which must include the simulated experience of administering and receiving physical restraint, instruction regarding the effects on the person restrained and on monitoring physical signs of distress, and more.
- Prone containment, which simultaneously immobilizes all four extremities, is prohibited except when used by trained personnel as a limited emergency intervention that is a documented part of a previously agreed upon written behavioral intervention plan. These rules do not limit school staff from using reasonable force to protect students, other persons or themselves from imminent, serious physical harm.
- Physical restraint may only be used when non-physical interventions would not be effective, the student's behavior poses a threat of imminent, serious, physical harm to self or others, and any applicable positive techniques from the student's behavioral intervention plan have been attempted. It is limited to the use of reasonable, necessary force. Physical restraint may not be used as a means of punishment or as an intervention designed or likely to cause physical pain. Only

trained personnel may administer restraints, and when possible it must be witnessed by at least one other adult who does not participate in the restraint. No restraint may prevent a student from breathing or speaking, and the student must be continuously monitored. The restraint must be released as soon as the student is no longer at risk of causing imminent physical harm to self or others. Each incident must be documented, there must be follow-up, and parents must be notified as soon as possible but no later than two school days later.

- Seclusion, placing a child alone in a locked room without supervision, is strictly prohibited. Seclusion is permitted when the student is under constant surveillance and observation and when documented as part of a previously agreed upon written behavioral intervention plan. Any intervention which denies adequate sleep, food, water, shelter, bedding or access to bathroom facilities is also prohibited.

South Carolina

None.

South Dakota

None.

Tennessee

Tenn. Code ann. §§ 49-10-1301 to -1306 (Education; Special Education; Special Education Isolation and Restraint Modernization and Positive Behavioral Supports Act)

- A special education student may only be restrained or isolated if the restraint or isolation is provided for in the student's IEP, or if there is an emergency and it is necessary to assure the physical safety of the student or others nearby. If an emergency situation, school personnel must immediately contact those school personnel designated to authorize the isolation or restraint, and they must evaluate the student's condition within a reasonable time. Parents must be notified the same day. Each incident must be documented. School personnel must remain in the physical presence of any restrained student and must continuously observe a student who is in isolation or being restrained to monitor the health and well-being of the student.

- As applied to special education students, chemical restraints are prohibited against unless under the direction of a physician and with parental consent; mechanical restraints are prohibited; and any form of life-threatening restraint, including restraint that restricts the flow of air into a person's lungs, is prohibited. Additionally, the use of isolation or physical restraint as a means of coercion, punishment, convenience, or retaliation is prohibited.
- Actions undertaken by school personnel to break up a fight or to take a weapon from a student are not prohibited.
- As applied to special education students, the use of a locked door or other structure that accomplishes the intent of locking a student in a room or structure, to isolate or seclude a student, is prohibited.

Texas

Tex. Educ. Code ann. § 37.002 1 (Education Code; Public Education; Safe Schools; Discipline, Law and Order; Alternative Settings for Behavior Management)

- Rules must be promulgated for the use of restraint and time-out by school personnel.
- Seclusion is a behavior management technique in which a student is confined in a locked space that is designed solely to seclude a person and contains less than 50 square feet of space. School personnel may not place a student in seclusion.
- This section does not prevent a student's locked, unattended confinement in an emergency situation while awaiting the arrival of law enforcement if the student possesses a weapon and the confinement is necessary to prevent bodily harm to the student or another person.

19 Tex. Admin. Code § 89.1053 (Education; Texas Education Agency; Adaptations for Special Populations; Commissioner's Rules Concerning Special Education Services; Clarification of Provisions in Federal Regulations and State Law)

- School personnel may only use restraint in an emergency in which a student's behavior poses a threat of imminent, serious physical harm to the student or others or imminent, serious property destruction. Restraint shall be limited to reasonable force as is necessary to address the emergency, shall be discontinued when the emergency no longer exists, shall be implemented as to protect the health and safety of the student, and shall not deprive the student of basic human necessities.
- A core team of school personnel must be trained in the use of restraint and must include special education personnel likely to use restraint. Personnel who use restraint but who have not received training must receive training within 30 days following the use of restraint. Training must include prevention and de-escalation techniques. Each incident must be documented, and parents must be notified the same day.
- Time-out is a behavior management technique in which the student is separated from other students in a setting that is not locked and from which the exit is not blocked. Physical force or threats may not be used to place a student in time-out. Time-out must be included in the student's IEP if it is utilized on a recurrent basis. School personnel must be trained in the use of time-out. Each instance must be documented.

Utah

Utah Code Ann. §§ 53a-11-801 to -806 (State System of Public Education; Students in Public Schools; Physical Restraint Guidelines)

- Corporal punishment is prohibited, unless the parents have provided written permission. However, corporal punishment does not include the use of reasonable and necessary physical restraint or force in self-defense, to obtain possession of a weapon or dangerous object, to protect the child or another person from physical injury, to remove from a situation a child who is violent or disruptive, or to protect property from damage.

- Behavior reduction intervention for students with disabilities is excepted from this part under certain circumstances.

Vermont

None.

Virginia

8 Va. Admin. Code § 20-670-130 (Education; State Board of Education; Regulation Governing the Operation of Private Day School for Students with Disabilities; Program Requirements)

- This section only applies to private day schools whose primary purpose is to provide educational services to persons with autism, developmental disabilities, deafness, mental retardation, emotional disturbance, learning disability or other certain disabilities. It does not apply to public schools or private day schools whose primary purpose is to provide educational services to students without disabilities, even though it may also serve children with disabilities.
- Parents must be informed of the policies of the school's behavior management or modification program, and informed consent must be obtained before implementation of any behavior management program.
- The use of physical restraints must follow written policies and procedures. Physical restraint is limited to that which is minimally necessary to protect the student or others and may only be used by trained staff after less intrusive interventions have failed and when failure to restrain would result in harm to students or others. Staff must review the training at least annually. Each incident must be documented and reported to the parents.
- Corporal punishment and the use of restraint as punishment, reprisal, or convenience is prohibited. The use of mechanical and chemical restraints is also prohibited.

Washington

Wash. Admin. Code 392-172a-03120 to -03135 (Superintendent of Public Instruction; Rules for the Provision of Special Education; Aversive Interventions)

- No school district may authorize or allow the use of aversive interventions on a special education student if the intervention would violate the conditions of this part.
- The use of force or restraint which is either unreasonable under the circumstances or deemed to be an unreasonable form of corporal punishment is prohibited. This includes interfering with a student's breathing, or physically restraining a student by binding or otherwise attaching the student's limbs together or by binding or otherwise attaching any part of the student's body to an object. However, this type is restraint is permissible if it is used when and to the extent reasonably necessary to protect the student, other persons, or property from serious harm. The restraint, including the duration of its use, must be provided for by the terms of the student's IEP. An adult must remain in visual or auditory range, and the student must either be capable of releasing himself or herself from the restraint, or must continuously remain within view of an adult.
- Aversive intervention does not include the use of reasonable force, restraint, or other treatment to control unpredicted spontaneous behavior which is a clear and present danger of serious harm to the student or another person, a clear and present danger of serious harm to property, or a clear and present danger of seriously disputing the educational process.
- Isolation, including the duration of its use, must be provided for by the terms of the student's IEP. The enclosure must be ventilated, lighted, temperature controlled, and permit continuous visual monitoring of the student from the outside. An adult must remain in visual or auditory range. The student must either be capable of releasing himself or herself from the enclosure, or must continuously remain within view of an adult.

West Virginia

W. Va. Code r. § 126-28-8 (Procedural Rule; West Virginia Board of Education; West Virginia's Universal Access to a Quality Early Education System)

- Staff members in a West Virginia pre-k classroom may not handle behavior problems by restraining a child by any means other than a firm grasp around a child's arms or legs and then for only as long as is necessary for the child to regain control.
- Staff members in a West Virginia Pre-k classroom may not handle behavior problems by isolating a child without supervision or placing the child in a dark area.

Wisconsin

None.

Wyoming

None.

GAO's Mission

The Government Accountability Office, the audit, evaluation, and investigative arm of Congress, exists to support Congress in meeting its constitutional responsibilities and to help improve the performance and accountability of the federal government for the American people. GAO examines the use of public funds; evaluates federal programs and policies; and provides analyses, recommendations, and other assistance to help Congress make informed oversight, policy, and funding decisions. GAO's commitment to good government is reflected in its core values of accountability, integrity, and reliability.

End Notes

[1] These are excerpts from the definitions used by the Centers for Medicare and Medicaid Services (CMS) and they apply to all hospitals participating in the Medicare and Medicaid programs. 42 C.F.R § 482. 13(e)(1)(i)-(ii). We chose to use the CMS definitions because there are no federal statutes that apply to seclusion or restraint in the context of public or private schools.

[2] GAO, *Mental Health: Extent of Risk from Improper Restraint or Seclusion is Unknown*, GAO/T-HEHS-00-026 (Washington, D.C.: Oct. 26, 1999).

[3] GAO, *Residential Treatment Programs: Concerns Regarding Abuse and Death in Certain Programs for Troubled Youth*, GAO-08-146T (Washington, D.C.: Oct. 10, 2007) and *Residential Programs: Selected Cases of Death, Abuse, and Deceptive Marketing*, GAO-08-713T (Washington, D.C.: Apr. 24, 2008).

[4] Arizona, Florida, Georgia, Idaho, Indiana, Kansas, Kentucky, Louisiana, Mississippi, Missouri, Nebraska, New Jersey, North Dakota, Oklahoma, South Carolina, South Dakota, Vermont, Wisconsin, and Wyoming.

[5] Alaska, Colorado, Hawaii, Michigan, Ohio, Utah, and Virginia.

[6] California, Colorado, Connecticut, Illinois, Iowa , Maine, Maryland, Massachusetts, Nevada, New Hampshire, New Mexico, New York, Oregon, Pennsylvania, Rhode Island, Texas, and Virginia.

[7] Colorado, Delaware, Maryland, Massachusetts, Montana, New Hampshire, New York, North Carolina, Oregon, Pennsylvania, Tennessee, Virginia, and Washington.

[8] California, Colorado, Connecticut, Illinois, Iowa, Maine, Maryland, Massachusetts, Minnesota, Nevada, New Mexico, New York, North Carolina, Oregon, Pennsylvania, Rhode Island, Tennessee, Texas, and Virginia.

[9] California and Connecticut.

[10] Colorado, Connecticut, Iowa, Massachusetts, Pennsylvania, Rhode Island, Tennessee, and Washington.

[11] There is likely a small percentage of overlapping allegations given our inability to reconcile information from the sources we used.

[12] For the purposes of this report, our definition of students with disabilities does not indicate eligibility under IDEA.

[13] Colorado, Delaware, Maryland, Massachusetts, Montana, New Hampshire, New York, North Carolina, Oregon, Pennsylvania, Tennessee, Virginia, and Washington.

[14] Colorado, Connecticut, Iowa, Massachusetts, Pennsylvania, Rhode Island, Tennessee, and Washington.

[15] California, Colorado, Connecticut, Illinois, Iowa , Maine, Maryland, Massachusetts, Nevada, New Hampshire, New Mexico, New York, Oregon, Pennsylvania, Rhode Island, Texas, and Virginia.

[16] At the time, this department was called the Department of Protective and Regulatory Services.

[17] The school implements a Behavior Support Plan in response to maladaptive and defiant behaviors by residents. The plan attempts to address and manage these behaviors; to foster more positive, appropriate, and pro-social behavior; and to ensure the safety of the residents and their peers.

In: Time Out: Examining Seclusion and... ISBN: 978-1-60876-932-2
Editor: Laura E. Kentley

Chapter 8

THE USE OF SECLUSION AND RESTRAINT IN PUBLIC SCHOOLS: THE LEGAL ISSUES*

Nancy Lee Jones and Jody Feder

SUMMARY

Seclusion and restraint have been used in various situations to deal with violent or noncompliant behavior. Because of recent congressional interest in the use of seclusion and restraint in schools, this report focuses on the legal issues concerning the use of these techniques in schools, including their application both to children covered by the Individuals with Disabilities Education Act (IDEA) and to those not covered by IDEA.

Several recent reports have documented instances of deaths and injuries resulting from the use of seclusion or restraints in schools, but there is no general reporting requirement so the exact parameters of the problem are unknown. On May 19, 2009, in conjunction with a hearing by the House Education and Labor Committee, the Government Accountability Office (GAO) released a study examining the use of seclusion and restraint in the education setting, finding hundreds of cases of alleged abuse and death due to the use of seclusion and restraint. On July 31, 2009, the Secretary of Education sent letters to Chief State School Officers noting the problems identified by the

---

* This is an edited, reformatted and augmented version of a CRS Report for Congress publication dated August 2009.

GAO report and in the May 19 congressional hearing, encouraging each state to review its current policies, and stating that the Chief State School Officers would be contacted by the Department of Education (ED) by August 15, 2009, to discuss relevant state laws, regulations, policies, and guidance. The results of these discussions are to be posted on ED's website.

Federal law does not contain general provisions relating to the use of seclusion and restraints, and there are no specific federal laws concerning the use of seclusion and restraint in public schools. The Individuals with Disabilities Education Act requires a free appropriate public education for children with disabilities, and an argument could be made that some uses of seclusion and restraint would violate this requirement. In addition, certain procedures may violate constitutional rights or state laws. Although there are some judicial cases, they do not provide clear guidance on when, if ever, seclusion and restraint may be used in schools.

INTRODUCTION

Seclusion and restraint have been used in various situations to deal with violent or noncompliant behavior. One of the most common settings for their use has been psychiatric hospitals,[1] but seclusion and restraint have also been used in other residential facilities[2] and in schools.[3] Because of recent congressional interest in the use of seclusion and restraint in schools,[4] this report focuses on the legal issues concerning the use of these techniques in schools, including their application both to children covered by the Individuals with Disabilities Education Act (IDEA)[5] and to those not covered by IDEA.

BACKGROUND

Several recent reports have documented instances of deaths and injuries resulting from the use of seclusion or restraints in schools but there is no general reporting requirement so the exact parameters of the problem are unknown.[6] On May 19, 2009, the Government Accountability Office (GAO), in conjunction with a hearing in the House Education and Labor Committee,[7] released a study examining the use of seclusion and restraint in the education setting, finding hundreds of cases of alleged abuse and death due to the use of seclusion and restraint.[8] GAO also examined state laws and noted that it "could not find a single Web site, federal agency, or other entity that collects information on the use of these methods or the extent of their alleged abuse."[9]

On July 31, 2009, the Secretary of Education sent letters to Chief State School Officers noting the problems identified by the GAO report and in the May 19 hearing in the House Education and Labor Committee.[10] The Secretary encouraged each state to review its current policies regarding the use of restraints and seclusion in schools and, if appropriate, develop or revise the policies prior to the start of the 2009-2010 school year. He noted the approach used in Illinois, which includes an emphasis on the use of positive behavior intervention and supports, and concluded by stating that the Chief State School Officers would be contacted by the Department of Education (ED) by August 15, 2009, to discuss relevant state laws, regulations, policies, and guidance. The results of these discussions are to be posted on ED's website.[11]

Federal law does not contain general provisions relating to the use of seclusion and restraints. However, certain uses of seclusion and restraints in health care facilities that receive federal funds and in certain non-medical, community-based facilities for children and youth are prohibited by the Children's Health Act of 2000.[12] In the 111th Congress, H.R. 911, a bill that would extend these rights to certain residential programs for children, passed the House on February 23, 2009,[13] and legislation regarding the use of seclusion and restraint in public and private schools may also be considered. Currently, there are no specific federal laws concerning the use of seclusion and restraint in public schools, although the Individuals with Disabilities Education Act requires a free appropriate public education for children with disabilities, and an argument could be made that some uses of seclusion and restraint would violate this requirement. In addition, certain procedures may violate constitutional rights or state laws.

Prior to examining legal principles involved in the use of seclusion and restraint in school, it is helpful to define the terms. Unfortunately, there is no specific federal statutory definition of the terms as used in school settings, although the terms have been defined in the context of community-based facilities for children and youth under the Children's Health Act of 2000.[14] For community-based facilities, seclusion is defined as the involuntary confinement of an individual alone in a room or an area from which the person is physically prevented from leaving.[15] Restraint is defined as a manual method, physical or mechanical device, material, or equipment, that immobilizes or reduces an individual's freedom of movement.[16]

CONSTITUTIONAL ISSUES

At times, the use of seclusion and restraint in public schools has been subject to constitutional challenge. Such challenges have primarily been based upon the Fourteenth Amendment's guarantee of due process and the Fourth Amendment's prohibition against unreasonable seizures, although other types of constitutional claims have been asserted at times.[17]

The Due Process clause of the Fourteenth Amendment prohibits the government from depriving an individual of his liberty without due process of the law.[18] Although the Supreme Court has not directly considered whether the use of seclusion and restraint in public schools violates the Due Process Clause, the Court has considered a related case involving restraint of a mentally retarded adult confined to a state hospital. In *Youngberg v. Romeo*,[19] the Court applied a reasonableness standard, holding that there is a constitutionally protected liberty interest in reasonably safe conditions of confinement and freedom from unreasonable bodily restraint. However, in order to determine what is reasonable, courts must defer to the judgment of qualified professionals.

In the public school setting, due process challenges to the use of seclusion and restraint have generally been rejected if such tactics are deemed to be reasonable, especially if such use constitutes a routine disciplinary technique. For example, in *Wallace by Wallace v. Bryant School District*, the court held that the plaintiff's isolation in a music room for three class periods was not a due process violation,[20] and in *Dickens v. Johnson County Board of Education*,[21] the court similarly rejected a due process challenge to a brief "timeout" imposed on a student because his seclusion "was not unduly harsh or grossly disproportionate."

In some cases, however, the use of seclusion and restraint may be actionable under the Due Process Clause if it is found to be unreasonable.[22] Courts are even more likely to find the use of seclusion and restraint to be unreasonable if such use is so extreme that it "shocks the conscience." Although many of these cases involve more extreme disciplinary methods, such as corporal punishment,[23] there have been some cases that involve seclusion and restraint. In *Orange v. County of Grundy*,[24] the court declined to dismiss a substantive due process claim, ruling that "placing school children in isolation [in a storage closet] for an entire school day without access to lunch or a toilet facility 'shocks the conscience.'" Indeed, the court emphasized that the use of seclusion must be reasonable, and school officials bear the responsibility to supervise students who are in isolation. Ultimately, however, the due process inquiry, and the reasonableness standard upon which it relies, are subjective and highly dependent on the facts in a given case, thus making it difficult to predict the outcome of a due process challenge to the use of seclusion and restraint in public schools.

Meanwhile, some plaintiffs have also claimed that the use of seclusion and restraint violates the Fourth Amendment, which prohibits the government from subjecting individuals to "unreasonable searches and seizures."[25] As with due process claims, courts assess such Fourth Amendment claims using a reasonableness standard.[26] For example, in Rasmus v. Arizona,[27] the court refused to dismiss a student's claim that his brief seclusion in a locked closet constituted a seizure in violation of the Fourth Amendment, reasoning that the seizure could be considered unreasonable because it violated the fire code and behavior management guidelines. In contrast, the court in *Couture v. Board of Education of the Albuquerque Public Schools* found that the use of supervised timeouts for a student who engaged in disruptive and threatening behavior was reasonable, particularly in light of the fact that the use of timeouts was authorized by the student's Individualized Education Plan (IEP).[28] Ultimately, like due process cases, the resolution of Fourth Amendment claims involving the use of seclusion and restraint generally depends on the facts of a given case, with a violation unlikely to be found except in cases involving excessive or unreasonable uses of such tactics.

Finally, it is important to note that constitutional claims have, in some cases, been limited by courts that may be reluctant to find constitutional violations for actions that could ordinarily be remedied under state tort law. For example, in Ingraham v. Wright, the Supreme Court acknowledged that "corporal punishment in public schools implicates a constitutionally protected liberty interest" under the Due Process Clause, but the Court nevertheless held that "the traditional common-law remedies are fully adequate to afford due process."[29] Thus, remedies for the unlawful use of seclusion and restraint should also be sought under state tort law.[30]

INDIVIDUALS WITH DISABILITIES EDUCATION ACT

Statutory Provisions

The Individuals with Disabilities Education Act (IDEA)[31] is the major federal statute for the education of children with disabilities. IDEA both authorizes federal funding for special education and related services[32] and, for states that accept these funds,[33] sets out principles under which special education and related services are to be provided. The requirements are detailed, especially when the regulatory interpretations are considered. The major principles include the following requirements:

- States and school districts make available a free appropriate public education (FAPE)[34] to all children with disabilities, generally between the ages of 3 and 21. States and school districts identify, locate, and evaluate all children with disabilities, regardless of the severity of their disability, to determine which children are eligible for special education and related services.
- Each child receiving services has an individual education program (IEP) spelling out the specific special education and related services to be provided to meet his or her needs. The parent must be a partner in planning and overseeing the child's special education and related services as a member of the IEP team.
- "To the maximum extent appropriate," children with disabilities must be educated with children who are not disabled; and states and school districts provide procedural safeguards to children with disabilities and their parents, including a right to a due process hearing, the right to appeal to federal district court, and, in some cases, the right to receive attorneys' fees.

IDEA provides that when the behavior of a child with a disability impedes the child's learning or the learning of others, the IEP team must consider "the use of positive behavioral interventions and supports, and other strategies, to address that behavior."[35] Nothing in IDEA specifically addresses the use of seclusion and restraints, and the Department of Education has stated that "[w]hile IDEA emphasizes the use of positive behavioral interventions and supports to address behavior that impedes learning, IDEA does not flatly prohibit the use of mechanical restraints or other aversive behavioral techniques for children with disabilities.[36] The Department also noted that state law may address whether restraints may be used and, if restraints are allowed, the "critical inquiry is whether the use of such restraints or techniques can be implemented consistent with the child's IEP and the requirement that IEP Teams consider the use of positive behavioral interventions and supports when the child's behavior impedes the child's learning or that of others."[37]

IDEA Judicial Decisions Involving Seclusion and Restraints

The Supreme Court has not specifically addressed the use of seclusion or restraints under IDEA; however, in *Honig v. Doe,*[38] the Court examined IDEA's requirements for children who exhibited violent or inappropriate behavior, and held that a suspension longer than 10 days violated IDEA's "stay-put" provision.[39] In *Honig*, the Court observed that this decision "does not leave educators hamstrung" and that educators may utilize "normal procedures" which "may include the use of study carrels, timeouts, detention, or the restriction of privileges" as well as a 1 0-day suspension.[40]

Despite the lack of specific language in IDEA regarding the use of restraints and seclusion, cases have been brought alleging that their use violates a child's right to a free appropriate public education.[41] In *Melissa S. v. School District of Pittsburgh,*[42] the Third Circuit addressed allegations of IDEA violations involving a school's response to the child's serious behavior problems. The court noted that the child "sat on the floor kicking and screaming, struck other students, spit at and grabbed the breast of a teacher, refused to go to class, and once had to be chased by her aide after running out of the school building."[43] In this situation, the school's use of a time-out area in an unused office where her aide and others would give her work and encourage her to go to class did not violate IDEA since it did not change the child's placement and was within normal procedures for dealing with children who were endangering themselves or others. Similarly, the Eighth Circuit in *CJN v. Minneapolis Public Schools*[44] held that a third grade child with brain lesions and a history of psychiatric illness received FAPE despite extensive use of seclusion since he was progressing academically and the school had made efforts to tailor his IEP to address his behavior. A strong dissent was filed, noting the child seemed to be trapped in an increasingly punitive approach to discipline,[45] and stating, "[w]e are essentially telling school districts that it's copacetic to deal with students with behavioral disabilities by punishing them for their disability, rather than finding an approach that addresses the problem. We also tacitly approve the District's resort to police intervention for the behavioral problems it helped create by failing to address CJN's unique behavioral disorder."[46]

Courts have examined whether the administrative exhaustion requirements of IDEA apply in situations involving the use of seclusion and restraint. In *C.N. v. Willmar Public Schools,*[47] the child's IEP and behavior intervention plan allowed for the use of seclusion and restraint procedures when the child was a danger to herself or others. The court required administrative exhaustion, finding that if the parent was dissatisfied with the child's education, she must follow the IDEA due process procedures and file for a due process hearing. Since the parent had not done so, the court dismissed the parent's complaint.[48] In a series of cases involving a special education teacher in Pennsylvania who allegedly hit, pinched, dragged, and restrained autistic students in Rifton chairs with bungee cords and/or duct tape, the district court originally did not require the exhaustion of administrative remedies.[49] However, the court later held that, due to a subsequent court of appeals decision mandating the use IDEA administrative procedures when a violation of FAPE was alleged, exhaustion was required and the IDEA claim was dismissed. This was despite the argument that the cases differed due to the physical and emotional abuse alleged in the lower court cases.[50]

In *Peters v. Rome City School District,*[51] although the child's mother had consented to the school's IEP which included use of a time-out room, the court found that this consent did not impact on her assertion of constitutional violations. The child's mother testified that she had not known how often the child had been placed in the room; how he was treated while there; and that the room was filthy and lacked ventilation. IDEA issues were not directly addressed in *Peters* since the school district had not objected to the court's failure to instruct the jury about the federal and state laws possibly allowing the use of time-out rooms.

In contrast, IDEA has been used by parents in an attempt to enjoin enforcement of a New York state regulation that banned the use of "aversive interventions."[52] Parents argued in part that "some students' IEP's were being revised without parental consent or simply not revised for the new school year, the effect of which was to deprive those students of aversive therapies."[53] The Second Circuit vacated the district court's injunction against the regulation and remanded for further findings, noting, "We are confident that, especially given the harms that could result if the student plaintiffs' behavioral treatments are interrupted, the deficiencies in the district court's order may be expeditiously remedied."[54]

State Laws and Policies

Several recent studies have examined state law and policies regarding seclusion and restraints in schools, and generally have found little uniformity in coverage. In a May 2009 study, GAO found that 19 states have no laws or regulations relating to the use of seclusion or restraints in schools, and that the states that have laws or regulations vary widely in their coverage.[55] For example, GAO found that 7 states have provisions restricting the use of restraints but do not regulate seclusion,[56] and 17 states require training prior to the administration of restraints.[57] A 2007 study which surveyed state educational agencies found that 24 states had an established policy or provided guidelines concerning the use of time-out procedures.[58] A January 2009 survey by the National Disability Rights Network examined the laws and policies of 56 states and territories and found that 41% had no laws or policies concerning restraint and seclusion, almost 90% allowed prone restraints,[59] and 45% required or recommended that schools notify parents or guardians of the use of restraints or seclusion.[60]

End Notes

[1] See Stacey A. Tovino, "Psychiatric Restraint and Seclusion: Resisting Legislative Solution," 47 Santa Clara L. Rev. 511 (2007).

[2] "Residential Facilities: State and Federal Oversight Gaps May Increase Risk to Youth Well-Being," Testimony of Kay E. Brown, GAO, Before the House Committee on Education and Labor (April 24, 2008).

[3] National Disability Rights Network, School is not Supposed to Hurt: Investigative Report on Abusive Restraint and Seclusion in Schools (January 2009) http://www.napas.org/sr/SR-Report.pdf.

[4] *Examining the Abusive and Deadly Use of Seclusion and Restraint in Schools: Hearings Before the House Comm. on Education and Labor,* 111th Cong. (2009), *http://edlabor.house.gov/hearings/2009/05/examining-the-abusive-anddead.shtml.*

[5] 20 U.S.C. § 1400 et seq.

[6] National Disability Rights Network, School is not Supposed to Hurt: Investigative Report on Abusive Restraint and Seclusion in Schools (January 2009) http://www.napas.org/sr/SR-Report.pdf. Protection & Advocacy, Inc., "Restraint & Seclusion in California Schools: A Failing Grade" (June 2007), http://www.disabilityrightsca.org/pubs/702301.pdf; Mark Sherman, "Lawmakers Discuss National Teacher Registry," 42 EDUCATION DAILY 1 (May 20, 2009).

[7] *Examining the Abusive and Deadly Use of Seclusion and Restraint in Schools: Hearings Before the House Comm. on Education and Labor,* 111th Cong. (2009), *http://edlabor.house.gov/hearings/2009/05/examining-the-abusive-anddead.shtml.*

[8] Government Accountability Office, *Seclusions and Restraints: Selected Cases of Death and Abuse at Public and Private Schools and Treatment Centers,*GAO-09-719T (May 19, 2009), http://www.gao.gov/new.items/d09719t.pdf.

[9] *Id.*

[10] http://www.ed.gov/policy/elsec/guid/secletter/090731.html.

[11] *Id.*

[12] P.L. 106-310, 42 U.S.C. §290ii.

[13] A similar bill, H.R. 6358, 1 10th Cong., passed the House on June 25, 2008, but was not considered in the Senate.

[14] P.L. 106-310, 42 U.S.C. §290ii.

[15] See 42 U.S.C. §290ii(d)(2), §290jj(d)(4); 42 C.F.R. §482. 13(e)(1)(ii). Various terms are sometimes used to describe related practices. One article has noted that in the educational setting the general term "timeout" can be divided into four types of interventions: (1) inclusion, (2) exclusion, (3) seclusion, and (4) restrained timeout. Inclusion timeouts are defined as the least restrictive and involved placing a student in a classroom area where she can observe the classroom but cannot participate in activities. Exclusion timeout is where a student is separated in a designated area away from his peers but is not prevented from leaving. Examples of exclusion timeouts include sitting in a corner of the classroom facing the wall or having a student place his head on his desk. Seclusion timeout is where a student is removed from the classroom environment, placed alone in a room, and prevented from leaving. Restrained timeout is a combination of use of timeout procedures and physical restraint. An example would be positioning a student in a chair in a corner and restraining the student from moving. Joseph B. Ryan, Reece L. Peterson, and Michael Rozalski, "State Policies Concerning the Use of Seclusion Timeout in Schools," 30 Education and Treatment of Children 215 (2007).

[16] See 42 U.S.C. §290ii(d)(1) §290jj(d)(1) and (2); 42 C.F.R. 482.13(e)(1)(i).

[17] See, e.g., Ingraham v. Wright, 430 U.S. 651 (1977) (holding that the Eighth Amendment's prohibition against cruel and unusual punishment was not applicable to corporal punishment inflicted by school administrators).

[18] U.S. Const. amend. XIV, § 1.

[19] 457 U.S. 307 (1982).

[20] 46 F. Supp. 2d 863, 867 (E.D. Ark. 1999).

[21] 661 F. Supp. 155 (E.D. Tenn. 1987).

[22] See, e.g., Jefferson v. Ysleta Independent School Dist., 817 F.2d 303 (5th Cir. Tex. 1987).

[23] See, e.g., Ingraham v. Wright, 430 U.S. 651 (1977); Neal v. Fulton County Bd. of Educ., 229 F.3d 1069 (1 1th Cir. Ga. 2000); Metzger v. Osbeck, 841 F.2d 518 (3d Cir. Pa. 1988); Hall v. Tawney, 621 F.2d 607 (4th Cir. W. Va. 1980). Physical restraint may rise to the level of corporal punishment, which involves physical pain inflicted upon the body, if such restraint is used as a form of physical punishment rather than as an educational or safety technique.

[24] 950 F. Supp. 1365 (E.D. Tenn. 1996).

[25] U.S. Const. amend. IV.

[26] N.J. v. T. L. O., 469 U.S. 325 (1985).

[27] 939 F. Supp. 709 (D. Ariz. 1996).

[28] 535 F.3d 1243 (10th Cir. N.M. 2008).

[29] Ingraham v. Wright, 430 U.S. 651, 672 (1977).

[30] Although public school officials may defend against such constitutional and tort claims by citing their qualified immunity from liability for the performance of official duties, that immunity is not available if the official violates a clearly established statutory or constitutional right of which a reasonable person would have had knowledge. Harlow v. Fitzgerald, 457 U.S. 800 (U.S. 1982). In some circumstances, however, state entities may be entitled to sovereign immunity under the Eleventh Amendment.

[31] 20 U.S.C. § 1400 et seq. For a more detailed discussion of IDEA see CRS Report RS22590, *The Individuals with Disabilities Education Act (IDEA): Overview and Selected Issues*, by Richard N. Apling and Nancy Lee Jones.

[32] Related services (for example, physical therapy) assist children with disabilities to help them benefit from special education (20 U.S.C. §1401(26)).

[33] Currently, all states receive IDEA funding.

[34] It should be emphasized that what is required under IDEA is the provision of a free appropriate public education. The Supreme Court, in *Board of Education of the Hendrick Hudson Central School District v. Rowley*, 458 U.S. 177 (1982), held that this requirement is satisfied when the state provides personalized instruction with sufficient support services to permit a child to benefit educationally from that instruction, and that this instruction should

be reasonably calculated to enable the child to advance from grade to grade. IDEA does not require that a state maximize the potential of children with disabilities.

[35] 20 U.S.C. §1414(d)(3)(B).

[36] Letter to Anonymous, 50 IDELR 228 (OSEP March 17, 2008). It should be noted that some definitions of restraints encompass the use of drugs as well as physical restraints. See 42 C.F.R. §482. 13(e)(1)(i). IDEA specifically prohibits schools from requiring a child to obtain certain medication. 20 U.S.C. §1412(a)(25).

[37] Letter to Anonymous, 50 IDELR 228 (OSEP March 17, 2008).

[38] 484 U.S. 305 (1988).

[39] Generally, IDEA requires that if there is a dispute between the school and the parents of a child with a disability, the child "stays put" in his or her current educational placement until the dispute is resolved using the due process procedures set forth in the statute. 20 U.S.C. §1415(j). For a more detailed discussion of Honig and the "stay put" provision see CRS Report RL32753, *Individuals with Disabilities Education Act (IDEA): Discipline Provisions in P.L. 1 08-446*, by Nancy Lee Jones.

[40] 484 U.S. 305, 325 (1988).

[41] In addition to the cases discussed subsequently, at least one case has been brought by a protection and advocacy agency seeking student records concerning the use of a seclusion room. The court denied access to the records. Wisconsin Coalition for Advocacy, Inc. v. State of Wisconsin Department of Public Instruction, 407F.Supp.2d 988 (W.D. Wisc. 2005).

[42] 183 Fed. Appx. 184 (3d Cir. 2006).

[43] *Id.* at 188.

[44] 323 F.3d 630 (8th Cir. 2003), cert. denied 540 U.S. 984 (2003).

[45] The dissent noted that the police had been called following an incident where the child pushed and kicked staff and threatened to kill them, and that the child's behaviors seemed to escalate with the increased use of seclusion until the child attempted to kill himself when in the locked seclusion room. The dissent also noted that when the child was placed by his mother in a private school where there was no locked seclusion or police intervention, the child's behavioral problems decreased and he showed an increased interest in learning, friends, and school.

[46] 323 F.3d 630, 649 (8th Cir. 2003).

[47] 2008 U.S .Dist. LEXIS 63673 (August 19, 2008).

[48] See also Doe v. S&S Consolidated I.S.D., 149 F.Supp.2d 274 (E.D. Texas 2001), where the court, in a case that also presented constitutional issues, dismissed the IDEA claims relating to restraints since IDEA's administrative procedures had not been exhausted.

[49] Vicky M. and Darin M. v. Northeastern Educational Intermediate Unit 19, 486 F. Supp.2d 437 (M.D. Pa. 2007); Kimberly F. v. Northeastern Educational Intermediate Unit 19, 2007 U.S. Dist. LEXIS 35778 (M.D. Pa. May 15, 2007); Eva L. v. Northeastern Educational Intermediate Unit 19, 2007 U.S. Dist. LEXIS 35787 (M.D. Pa. May 15, 2007); John G. and Gloria G. v. Northeastern Educational Intermediate Unit 19, 2007 U.S. Dist. LEXIS 35786 (M.D. Pa. May 15, 2007); Sanford D. v. Northeastern Educational Intermediate Unit 19, 2007 U.S. Dist. LEXIS 35776 (M.D. Pa. (May 15, 2007); Joseph M. v. Northeastern Educational Intermediate Unit 19, 516 F.Supp.2d 424 (M.D. Pa. (2007); Thomas R. v. Northeastern Educational Intermediate Unit 19, 2007 U.S. Dist. LEXIS 8017 (M.D. Pa. (May 15, 2007).

[50] Vicky M. and Darin M. v. Northeastern Educational Intermediate Unit 19, 2007 U.S. Dist. LEXIS 71406 (M.D. Pa. September 26, 2007); Kimberly F. v. Northeastern Educational Intermediate Unit 19, 2007 U.S. Dist. LEXIS 71394 (M.D. Pa. September 26, 2007); Eva L. v. Northeastern Educational Intermediate Unit 19, 2007 U.S. Dist. LEXIS 71425 (M.D. Pa. September 26, 2007); John G. and Gloria G. v. Northeastern Educational Intermediate Unit 19, 2007 U.S. Dist. LEXIS 71365 (M.D. Pa. September 26, 2007); Sanford D. v. Northeastern Educational Intermediate Unit 19, 2007 U.S. Dist. LEXIS 71413 (M.D. Pa. (September 26, 2007); Joseph M. v. Northeastern Educational Intermediate Unit 19, 2007

U.S. Dist. LEXIS 71410 (M.D. Pa. September 26, 2007); Thomas R. v. Northeastern Educational Intermediate Unit 19, 2007 U.S. Dist. LEXIS 71416 (M.D. Pa. September 26, 2007).

[51] 747 N.Y. S.2d 867 (NYSC 2002).

[52] Alleyne v. New York State Education Department, 516 F.3d 96 (2d Cir. 2008). Aversive interventions were defined as including "skin shocks, 'contingent' food programs, and physical restraints." *Id.* at 98.

[53] *Id.* at 99.

[54] *Id.* at 102.

[55] Government Accountability Office, *Seclusions and Restraints: Selected Cases of Death and Abuse at Public and Private Schools and Treatment Centers,*GAO-09-7 19T (May 19, 2009), http://www.gao.gov/new.items/d09719t.pdf. GAO identified these states as Arizona, Florida, Georgia, Idaho, Indiana, Kansas, Kentucky, Louisiana, Mississippi, Missouri, Nebraska, New Jersey, North Dakota, Oklahoma, South Carolina, South Dakota, Vermont, Wisconsin, and Wyoming.

[56] *Id.* GAO identified the states that place restrictions on the use of restraints but not seclusions as Alaska, Colorado, Hawaii, Michigan, Ohio, Utah, and Virginia.

[57] *Id.* GAO identified the states that require training as California, Colorado, Connecticut, Illinois, Iowa , Maine, Maryland, Massachusetts, Nevada, New Hampshire, New Mexico, New York, Oregon, Pennsylvania, Rhode Island, Texas, and Virginia.

[58] Joseph B. Ryan, Reece L. Peterson, and Michael Rozalski, "State Policies Concerning the Use of Seclusion Timeout in Schools," 30 Education and Treatment of Children 215 (2007).

[59] Prone restraint is considered to have serious potential risks, including suffocation. See Protection and Advocacy, Inc., "The Lethal Hazard of Prone Restraint: Positional Asphyxiation" (April 2002), http://www.pai-ca.org/pubs/ 701801.pdf.

[60] National Disability Rights Network, School is not Supposed to Hurt: Investigative Report on Abusive Restraint and Seclusion in Schools (January 2009), http://www.napas.org/sr/SR-Report.pdf. The California legislature passed legislation, S.B. 1515, limiting the use of seclusion and restraint, but this bill was vetoed by the governor on September 29, 2008. It is interesting to note that one recent reported situation indicates that laws prohibiting the use of restraints and seclusion may result in increased police involvement. See Christina E. Sanchez, "Autistic Boy's Arrest at School Fuels Debate on Discipline for Disabled" (March 29, 2009), http://www.tennessean.com/article/20090329/NEWS04/ 9032903 70/1006/NEWS0 1.

INDEX

E

F

N

O

P

R

S

T